I'm Going to Be a Dad!

The Ultimate Pregnancy Handbook for First-Time Fathers: How to Become the Best Partner — Pregnancy Tips and Insights for Excited Dads-To-Be

David Hall

Contents

Introduction

Congratulations, Dad!

There's nothing that can beat the internal excitement of knowing you are expecting a child. The anticipation (that is also largely mixed with fear) you feel is unmatched by any other life event and if it's your first child, you're probably a gigantic ball of anxiety. Let me start by giving you a metaphorical pat on the back and offering congratulations for making a human being. Perhaps you are on the precipice of fatherhood, or perhaps this is not your first rodeo; the fact is, there is still a buzz of expectation surrounding the arrival of the baby.

Congratulations to you, Dad! Or Papa, Baba or Daddy, depending on what is acceptable in your society as a name for the male parent. This is a name you should get used to being called for the rest of your life, because fatherhood does not end. From the time that that baby is ejected from the birth canal, kicking and screaming, you'll be their dad. When they get a 100° fever and they have thrown up all over the kitchen floor, you'll be their dad. When they graduate high school and decide not to go to college, you'll still be their dad. No matter the path they choose for their life, you will always be their dad.

It is such a special role. It is a unique role. A father is like a real-life super-hero who is there to guide, protect, and have fun with. A father teaches their children life skills that they learned in their life. A father is your first friend. That is the role you are stepping into now. It can be overwhelming thinking about how much you will be to one small person or several little people. The good news is that the role is so fulfilling; when they smile and throw their little hands around your neck to kiss you is all the payment you need for this demanding role.

You are in for a wild ride. As an expectant father, you may not do the heavy lifting when it comes to the biological legwork of making the baby, but it does not excuse you from any heavy lifting at all. You have to involve yourself in every aspect of the pregnancy in order to feel connected to it. You need to be as involved as the parent who is carrying the baby in their body. She is not pregnant; you are both pregnant. This is your journey as well, and there is only one requirement: Be involved.

When You're Expecting, Expect This

You need to take the next nine months seriously. Because you are getting involved and not taking a back seat, you have to be prepared. You are not playing the dad who only purchases food cravings and tags along to obstetrician appointments. Expect the worst and plan for it. You have to think about the health benefits of the mother of the child and how that will affect your baby. You have to think about money, if there will be enough of it when the baby arrives.

Nowadays the relationship between parents is not as traditional if you compare it to a decade ago. Some couples are not married, by choice, when they conceive. Some are. Some couples are in a gray area. The relationship status between you and the mother of the child will dictate a lot. Pregnancy comes pre-packed with its own emotional rollercoaster, and as the parents, you have a front row seat. In spite of this, you have to soldier on. Remember that you are here to provide support during pregnancy and give love to your child, no matter what.

Over the next nine months, you have to think about where the baby will sleep; will they have a nursery? Do you have to move in with the mother? Is the relationship between the two of you strained? Who will pay for the birth? Who will stay and care for the baby after birth? These are all the logistical issues you will have to deal with as a father. You have to worry about it. You're not allowed to let your partner worry about anything, they have the job of making the baby; everything else is on you.

Expect the journey to be hard, yet rewarding. Expect difficult conversations that need to be had in order for things to be smoothed out before the baby arrives. Expect the expectant mother to get frustrated every step of the way. Expect moments of joy that bring tears to your eyes. Expect to be scared. Expect to be the worst and best versions of yourself. Expect to do more; expect to do everything.

My Mistakes

I made the unfortunate decision to take a back seat during my wife's first pregnancy. I was young and all the books I read about pregnancy made it seem like there was nothing much I could do but attend appointments and pay for everything. After the baby came, my wife sat me down and told me that if we were blessed with more children, I would have to be more hands-on. The second and third time around, I did not miss a beat. I was attentive and paid attention to the details. My wife now uses me as an example to tell her girlfriends what is, and is not, acceptable.

For me to become the standard, I had to make some regrettable mistakes. Luckily, I made those mistakes so that you don't have to. Pregnancy is not a "woman thing." If you helped in the conception of that baby, it's your thing too. I was not as dependable as I should have been; I could have been better at the little things. I trusted the hospital, my mother, and mother-in-law to make sure my wife was okay. I delegated a job only suited to me and man; oh, do I wish I could have those moments back.

Due to my nonchalance, my wife's stress levels were high. By herself, she had to figure out a lot of the logistics of the birth and what was supposed to happen. I don't think I even remember how the birth plan was conceived, although I did know it back to front. Can you see how terrible that looks? My wife had the gargantuan task of making a baby, yet also having to figure out all these other things alone, while my life barely changed.

I'm ashamed of how I behaved, but I learned the hard way what the word "father" means. Your job begins before the baby arrives, and will continue until your last breath. Lean into it with all that you have. Be enthusiastic and present in every moment. Understand that, once the time has passed, you will never get it back again.

Be Kind

You will never truly understand what it's like to be pregnant, but you can try to be empathetic. This book will be your guide throughout the pregnancy so you can stay in the loop of what is happening to mom and baby and what you should be doing. Be patient and kind, no matter which pregnancy stage you are in. Mom is doing the best she can and you have to do the best you can. Pregnancy is a special time; it's not always rainbows and butterflies, but it can be smooth sailing for both of you if you support one another. You have to put in the work.

In the next chapter, we will dissect how the conception happened and further discuss the first few weeks of pregnancy. You may be amazed at the miracle of conception; so many factors have to be perfectly aligned for pregnancy to occur. The way the baby forms in those crucial moments is also something that is awe-inspiring, and I will spare no details. Congratulations again Dad, you're in for quite a wild ride!

Chapter 1
First Trimester
(Conception to 4 Weeks)

Somehow, fate has smiled upon you and your partner, and you're bringing a little one into the world. At this point though, the expectant mom may not be aware of what is happening, because they may not be aware that they have missed a period. You may be asking yourself when pregnancy actually begins, and that's a wonderful question. For me to answer it, I have to start from the very beginning.

For conception to occur, an adult male and female need to have had sexual intercourse where the male ejaculates semen into the female's vagina. It sounds very simple, yet it is very complicated. Let's go through the prerequisites first before we break down the actual moment of conception. I thought I knew a lot about making a baby, only to find out I actually did not know that much. This chapter will be a step-by-step explanation of what it takes to make a baby.

But First, Puberty

"Puberty is a key stage in the transition from childhood to adulthood. It is a normal part of growing up, and each person's experience of it is unique" (Brazier, 2020). Both males and females have to transition into adulthood before they have the capability to make a baby. Basically, during puberty, levels of hormones like testosterone (for males) and estrogen (for females) begin to increase, which results in various changes in the body.

For males, typical signs of puberty include the testicles and penis increasing in size; hair will begin to grow on the pubic area, the face, armpits, chest, and back. The larynx will also grow, which will result in a low-pitched, deeper voice; sometimes the voice cracks and the Adam's apple also increases in size. Males going through puberty may experience growth spurts and, more significantly, they may also experience wet dreams, ejaculation during sleep, and spontaneous erections.

For females going through puberty, the typical signs are developing a breast bud, experiencing a period, and pre-menstrual syndrome. Depending on where they are in their menstrual cycle, females may have fluctuating hormones. Other signs of puberty include hair growing on the legs, underarms, and pubic area. Depending on the body, the hips may even widen and the waist may shrink in size, while the belly and buttock area increase in size. Due to genetics and other factors, everyone will develop at their own pace and in different ways.

Once puberty has occurred, it is likely that a person will have the functioning tools to make a baby without medical intervention. If an adult man has a functioning penis that is able to ejaculate a healthy semen sample that includes healthy sperm cells into the vaginal canal of an adult woman during sexual intercourse whilst the woman is ovulating, there is a high chance of conception.

Conception and How All of That Happened

So, aside from the sex part, how was the baby actually made? For a baby to be successfully conceived, four things have to have occurred. Firstly, the sperm should be transported to the egg; secondly, ovulation has to occur, and the egg should be transported to the fertilization site (fallopian tube); thirdly, the egg should be fertilized by the sperm, and lastly, the fertilized egg should successfully implant in the lining of the uterus and continue to develop. I know it sounds like I went from 0–100 with the terminology, but it's less complicated than it sounds.

Sperm Delivery

There are some prerequisites that should occur if the sperm should arrive successfully at the fertilization site. The sperm should be able to propel itself past the vagina and cervix, and have the ability to convert into the form of itself that can properly merge with the membrane on the outer layer of the egg. The transportation of sperm is not only dependent on the physical capability of the sperm, but also on the environment the sperm is being released into. The vagina and uterus need to be in a condition that is favorable to the survival of the sperm.

After ejaculation, semen is covered in a gel that will protect it from the acidic nature of the vagina, so that it is protected as it travels toward the egg. The cervical mucus that protects the entrance of the uterus becomes a haven for sperm during ovulation, as its PH changes to aid sperm survival. After sperm have successfully passed through the cervix and are now in the uterus, they will be swimming toward the fallopian tubes with the assistance of small uterine contractions.

It is estimated that sperm takes a few minutes to reach the fallopian tube following ejaculation. It is not always first come, first serve, and the first sperm to arrive at the egg is unlikely to be the fertilizing sperm. If the conditions are right, sperm can survive in the fallopian tubes for up to five days.

Ovulation

In order for the egg to be transported to the fallopian tube, ovulation has to occur. This transportation of the egg begins during ovulation and will end when the egg has reached the uterus. On the end of the fallopian tubes, there are tiny finger-like tubes that will sweep over the ovary in order to pick up an egg with its cilia; due to them being adhesive, the cilia are responsible for ensuring that the egg is picked up from the ovary and moved into the fallopian tube. The cilia and the contractions create a forward motion that move the egg along.

Egg transport from the ovary and through the fallopian tube takes roughly 30 hours. This is why couples may take some time to conceive.

There is no way to predict when exactly that egg will be there waiting, therefore you are unable to be accurate with your sperm transportation. You have to use various tools to estimate as best you can so that the sperm finds a healthy egg waiting for it. Damage to the fallopian tubes due to conditions like endometriosis or pelvic infection can cause scarring that prevents the proper functioning of the tubes.

Fertilization

Once the egg is moved from the ovary to the fallopian tubes, the fertilization window is only open from 12–24 hours. Fertilization is the union of the sperm with the egg. There is no guarantee that contact with sperm will result in fertilization of the egg, as this contact is random and unpredictable. There is a section of the fallopian tube (the ampullary-isthmic junction) where the egg will rest for around 30 hours, and this is where the fertilization occurs. Once the egg is fertilized, it will begin to descend to the uterus at an accelerated pace.

The reason for the 30-hour rest period is to ensure that the fertilized egg is properly developed as it begins its descent to the uterus. This time is also used for the uterus to prepare for the implantation of the egg into the uterus lining. If there are issues surrounding transport of the fertilized egg, it may result in an ectopic/tubal pregnancy, which is a pregnancy that results when a fertilized egg transplants into the fallopian tube. The fallopian tube is not an ideal place for a developing pregnancy, as there is no space in the tube; failure to identify an ectopic pregnancy may lead to a ruptured tube, which is dangerous to the woman.

There is a special membrane that surrounds the egg called the zona pellucida. This membrane is important because it serves two functions, namely: It has sperm receptors that allow sperm to fertilize the egg; and, once this fertilization happens, the zona pellucida ensures no other sperm can penetrate the egg, as it becomes impenetrable. After the sperm cell has penetrated the egg, cell division begins, and it is referred to as an embryo.

Implantation

As the embryo descends to the uterus, the cells are dividing continuously until it reaches the stage where it is referred to as a blastocyst. An embryo becomes a blastocyst five to six days after fertilization has occurred; it then sheds the zona pellucida so that it can begin implanting in the wall of the uterus. Just because an embryo is on track development-wise does not mean it will implant successfully. Even when the embryo implants successfully, cell division may stop. In both cases, the pregnancy would have ended. The uterus must be receptive to the implantation of the embryo, and the embryo itself must have the capability to attach itself successfully.

What's Happening to Baby

Technically, during week one and two there is no pregnancy, as it is the beginning of the woman's cycle. Week two is when ovulation happens, and week three begins the development of the baby. After fertilization, the one cell structure is referred to as a zygote, which then quickly develops into a ball of cells called a blastocyst. At this stage, the size of the embryo is about the same size as the head of a pin. It is at this stage that the embryo can split into two, thus resulting in identical twins.

Fraternal twins may also occur in the third week of pregnancy; they differ from identical twins in that identical twins come from one egg and one sperm, while fraternal twins come from two eggs and two sperm, due to more than one egg being released during fertilization. Identical twins are much rarer than fraternal twins. During this time, the embryo is developing and seeking to implant in the uterus so that it is able to develop into a healthy baby over the next 37 weeks.

During week four, implantation occurs. The growing embryo will burrow into the lining of the uterine wall and attach itself firmly. The attachment of the embryo to the uterus signals to the woman's body not to shed the lining, as there is a viable pregnancy. As the cells within the embryo continue to divide, the inner cells are what will develop into your baby, and the outer cells begin to form what will become the placenta.

What's Happening to Mom

At the end of week three or beginning of week four, there is a possibility of experiencing implantation spotting. The burrowing of the embryo into the lining of the uterus has consequences; it may cause a small bleed due to the blood vessels present on the uterine wall. Not every woman will experience implantation bleeding. It is important to note that this kind of bleeding is very light, short, occurs six to ten days after ovulation, and can be mistaken for the beginning of a period.

In week four, a woman may experience the same kind of PMS symptoms she goes through every month before she gets her period. This includes, but is not limited to, fatigue, bloating, mood fluctuations, cramps, and tenderness in the breasts. Early pregnancy signs are often similar to, or the same as, the symptoms Mom may experience before a period; that is why she may be pregnant, but think it is business as usual. The only way to confirm suspicion of a pregnancy is for the woman to take a pregnancy test.

What You Should Do

Sometimes pregnancies are happy accidents, and other times they have been planned to the last detail. If you are actively trying to have a baby, use this time to plan some dates in order to distract you from the two-week wait of wondering whether or not conception has happened and if it will result in a successful pregnancy. You may be as anxious as she is to find out whether or not she is pregnant, so you both may need activities to soothe this anxiety and bring you closer as a couple. Plan something that you will both enjoy; let your partner know how much you appreciate them.

Be excited if your partner has already started to think she's pregnant. Mirror her reactions. If she's unsure about how she feels, reassure her that no matter what she feels, you will be there to support her. I may have messed up my first time, but I know I just had to be there; do the same. Pregnancy can make a woman feel very alone, as the physical changes happen only to her. Reassure her she is not alone. Think about buying some pregnancy tests in order to confirm the pregnancy first at home. She may need to "pee on a few sticks" before she gets the positive that she suspects she is. Be a calming force and hold her hand every step of the way.

Volunteer to set up the first doctor's appointment with an obstetrician. This is ultimately the person who may deliver your baby. Sometimes your partner's obstetrician is also her gynecologist, so just have a discussion on the person she may want to go and see. They will likely repeat a pregnancy test and do an ultrasound in order to see what's happening with the baby, and also date the pregnancy by measuring the baby. You will receive your EDD (expected due date) at this first appointment.

Ensure that your partner is taking the right nutritional supplements or is eating a healthy diet. Encourage her to incorporate some physical exercise into her schedule, as well as setting some time apart to rest in order to lessen the fatigue and mood fluctuation symptoms. A lot of people lead busy lives, but when you are responsible for creating a life within you, you should also give your body time to rest from a grueling schedule. If there are things that you can do to lighten her load, then you should offer to do them.

What You Should Not Do

Waiting to find out whether or not your partner is pregnant can bring a lot of anxiety and stress into the relationship. This is especially true for couples that may have been trying to conceive for a long period of time. Do not obsess over whether or not your partner is pregnant, as this may place undue pressure on her. Take every day as it comes, and take a pregnancy test once she has missed her period.

There are some women that may get a positive pregnancy test in the third week, but it is recommended that you wait until your partner has missed their period before taking a pregnancy test. Do not force your partner to take a pregnancy test before she has missed her period, as this may be too early. Pregnancy tests are designed to detect human chorionic gonadotropin (hCG), and it is often undetectable in week three. Follow the rule of thumb and only encourage your partner to pee on that stick when her period is AWOL.

In the next chapter, we will be discussing the initial weeks of her pregnancy and what those look like for your baby and the mom. During this stage, the embryo is rapidly developing and quickly becoming a recognizable baby. Unfortunately for your partner, this may be the time where morning sickness kicks in and the pregnancy symptoms develop. What will be outlined in the next chapter will not only give you information on how the baby is developing, but also what you can do to assist your partner in getting through the initial changes.

The changes that accompany pregnancy can be jarring, especially if it is your first child. There is so much you cannot predict and will have to deal with as the pregnancy is unfolding. Your partner is as terrified as you. You both have no idea what pregnancy symptoms your partner will experience, or even if the pregnancy will have a happy ending. In order to cope, Dad, you should take it one day at a time.

Chapter 2
First Trimester (5–8 Weeks)

The pregnancy is in its infancy, but there is a lot that is going on. Big changes happen to both the pregnant woman and the baby she is carrying. You will also be inevitably excited during this time, as this is when you are probably looped into what is suspected. This is where people think the pregnancy begins, although it began around two or three weeks ago. This time is where most women receive a positive pregnancy test, because they inevitably missed their period.

The baby is very small, but there are a lot of big changes that are happening to them, as well as your partner. Receiving the news that a baby is coming may throw the both of you into a tailspin of emotions. It is natural to feel happy and scared at the same time. You may even begin to doubt your competence as a father: Do you really have the capability to be a good father, or is this baby doomed along with you? Every father has gone through this phase of being happy that they are about to become a father, yet also wondering if they will be a good father.

The fact that you are even worrying if you will be a good father shows that you are probably going to be a great one. But before we get to the value you bring as a father, let us make sure you bring the right kind of value as a partner to a pregnant woman. Unfortunately, this is also a very terrifying time for Mom, because she is also at risk of experiencing a loss. Not all pregnancies will end happily; there is a higher risk for miscarriage in the first trimester than in the second and third trimester. Your partner may never experience a loss, but they occur quite often; therefore, it is better to discuss why they happen and how to deal with them. I would prefer you had the information and not need it, rather than needing it and not having it.

Dealing With Loss

No one thinks that they have to deal with a loss until reality is staring them in the face. This is a difficult thing to deal with, whether you expected it or not. When you receive the news that your partner is pregnant, you are filled with excitement and hope for the future; you may even daydream with your partner about the sex of the baby and what your future as parents may look like. These dreams may be dashed when your partner experiences a miscarriage. Knowing how to deal with that disappointment and pain may be essential to your healing process as a couple.

Miscarriage, which is also referred to as spontaneous abortion, is characterized by the loss of a pregnancy before 20 weeks of gestation. "The American College of Obstetricians and Gynecologists (ACOG) estimates it is the most common form of pregnancy loss. It is estimated that as many as 26% of all pregnancies end in miscarriage and up to 10% of clinically recognized pregnancies" (Dugas & Slane, 2019). This is not a topic that is widely discussed, but it is not uncommon for a woman to experience a miscarriage in early pregnancy.

A woman may experience a chemical pregnancy and not even know it. This type of pregnancy accounts for a large percentage of the miscarriages that occur. A chemical pregnancy is where a pregnancy is lost shortly after implantation and passes via bleeding that occurs around the time that she receives her monthly period. Numerous women are unaware of the fact that they may have conceived and take the bleeding as a normal period, when in fact, it is the culmination of a chemical pregnancy.

Causes and Signs of Miscarriage

The cause of miscarriage in early pregnancy could be due to a number of things, but it is commonly attributed to chromosomal abnormalities. Other causes that can lead to miscarriage include infection, abnormalities in the uterus, the age of the woman, improper implantation, et cetera. No matter the cause of a miscarriage, you should be aware of the warning signs so that you know when to seek medical care for your partner. Signs of a miscarriage may include the following:

- heavy bleeding
- intense back pain
- white/pink mucous from the vagina
- sudden decline in pregnancy symptoms
- tissue/clots passing from the vagina

Types of Miscarriage

There are different kinds of miscarriages to consider, as it is often not a singular event, but rather a process that your partner may go through. A threatened miscarriage is when there is some bleeding during early pregnancy that is accompanied by cramps or backache. In this case, the cervix is closed and the bleeding may be attributable to implantation. An incomplete miscarriage, which is also referred to as an inevitable miscarriage, occurs when the cramps are accompanied by bleeding and the cervix is open.

A complete miscarriage is when the uterus is empty and the embryo and its tissue have been expelled via the vagina. Once this emptying is complete, the cramping and bleeding should subside. A complete miscarriage is confirmed by an ultrasound that is performed by your obstetrician or after you undergo surgical curettage. A missed miscarriage occurs when the embryo has died (no fetal heartbeat), but for some reason the embryo is not expelled, nor is there any bleeding. A recurrent miscarriage can occur if a woman has experienced three or more miscarriages that have taken place in the first trimester. This affects only about 1% of couples that are trying for a baby.

Prevention and Treatment of Miscarriage

Due the fact that a majority of miscarriages are caused by chromosomal abnormalities, there is not much your partner can do in order to prevent them. The only thing that can be vital when trying to conceive a healthy baby is to ensure that both you and your partner are in good health. Before you think about conceiving, you should ensure that you and your partner are eating healthy and balanced meals, that you both partake in regular exercise, that you both maintain a healthy weight, that neither of you abuse drugs or alcohol, and that you both take folic acid daily.

When you receive the good news that your partner is with child, you can take extra precautions to ensure you maintain their good health. When she has provided a healthy environment for the baby to grow, the pregnancy is more likely to thrive. Ensure that your partner keeps their abdomen safe and that they do not expose themselves to alcohol, secondhand smoke, caffeine, or radiation, and that they don't partake in contact sports or dangerous activities. Keeping your partner healthy and safe will increase the likelihood of her carrying the pregnancy to term.

Treatment for a miscarriage will depend on the kind of miscarriage that has occurred; the doctor will recommend the best course of action. Aside from the physical treatment of a miscarriage, it is also necessary to address the emotional consequences that may occur. Couples that miscarry have essentially experienced a loss of life and will need to grieve this loss. You and your partner will be left with a lot of unanswered questions as to why it happened and if your partner will be able to conceive again. Be open and honest with your partner about your feelings and allow her to express hers. If you need additional support, let your healthcare provider know. You can also lean on your faith and support groups online during this difficult time.

What's Happening to Baby

At five weeks, your baby is about the size of a strawberry seed. In spite of their small size, they are growing at an accelerated rate. The brain and the heart are beginning to form and the embryo is starting to look like a tadpole because of the neural tube that begins at the top of the embryo and ends at the bottom of it. The embryo is dividing cells to make three layers: the ectoderm (outer) layer that will become the nervous system, and the baby's hair, nails and skin; the mesoderm (middle) layer that will become the circulatory system and aid in developments of baby's heart, bones, blood, kidneys, and muscles; and the endoderm (inner) layer that will develop into the baby's liver, intestines, and lungs. The gestational sac forms around week five as well.

At six weeks, your baby is now the size of a grain of rice. Two major developments are unfolding during this week: The baby's heart begins to beat, and the neural tube closes. The baby's optic ventricle has fully formed and will become the eyes. The nose, jaw, and ears are taking form, and the limb buds that will develop into arms and legs are showing. In early development are the baby's urinary, reproductive, and digestive systems. At seven weeks, the baby is about the size of a blueberry and the ears, eyes, nose, and mouth are looking a lot more defined.

With the development of the eyelids and the tongue, week seven also sees the umbilical cord coming to life; the cord is a lifeline from the baby to the placenta, transferring oxygen and nutrients from the placenta to the baby and carrying waste from the baby. As your baby continues to develop, their kidneys also go through several developmental stages. It is likely that in the seventh week of pregnancy, the embryo has gotten to their second set of kidneys, but they are still in development.

At eight weeks, your baby will be around the size of a kidney bean and they will be looking more human than in the previous weeks. At this stage, the baby's body will begin to look less like a tadpole as the embryonic tail disappears and the limb buds extend. Tiny fingers and toes are developing within the limbs. As the digestive system develops, there is little room inside the embryo for the intestines, so they spill into the umbilical cord. When the baby has developed enough and there is more space in their abdomen, the intestines will move from the umbilical cord to the baby's abdomen.

The baby's facial features are also becoming more defined. What is note-worthy in week eight is that the reproductive organs are in full development as well, although they are not yet visible. Testes or ovaries are being formed, but you and your partner will not get to see them or find out the gender of the baby until they have reached around 20 weeks of gestation. The baby's bean-like appearance on an ultrasound is quite amusing to most parents, and it is common for them to nickname the baby "bean."

What's Happening to Mom

At week five, your partner may experience a missed period, tender or tingly breasts, increased fatigue, increased urination, mood swings, and morning sickness. Pregnancy symptoms vary depending on the woman. Some may have the worst of it and others will experience nothing at all. During week six, these symptoms may intensify because of the increased levels of hCG and progesterone in expectant mom's body. Her body may do its best to adjust to these changes, but the increased progesterone will lead to more fatigue. Your partner's doctor may do an ultrasound at six weeks in order to verify the pregnancy, check if there is only one baby, and check if there is a heartbeat. This will be an exciting time where you may get to see your baby and take a picture of the ultrasound home with you.

In the seventh week of pregnancy, there are a lot of changes that involve the cervix. In order to ensure the baby is safe within its mother's uterus, the cervix plays a pivotal role by remaining closed until the baby is ready to be born. Before the woman goes into labor, the cervix cannot dilate or efface; therefore, a mucus plug has to form. The mucus plug develops as a result of increased hormones and blood flow; leukorrhea (milky-white, odorless, thin discharge) clumps together to create a seal at the entrance of the uterus. This mucus plug also prevents bacteria from entering the uterus and harming the baby.

Constipation is something the expectant mom should expect to experi-ence due to the increased levels of progesterone. She may also experience bloating and gas. Progesterone makes the intestines move much slower than normal, meaning more water is absorbed from food waste and the stools inevitably become firmer. A pregnant woman's sense of smell becomes sharpened after conception, as it is believed it assists her in avoiding danger; unfortunately, this sharpened sense of smell can also wreak havoc on morning sickness and make her life hell.

At eight weeks pregnant, your partner will be two months pregnant and two-thirds of the way into her first trimester. The growth of the uterus may cause your partner to feel cramps; if they are not consistent or intense in pain, they are usually nothing to worry about. She may also experience more breast changes, where you both may "notice veins on the surface skin of her breasts as more blood flows to the area, the nipple and areola may get darker, and her breast may feel full and sore" (Pevzner, 2021f). If the pregnancy symptoms are getting the better of your partner, make sure she considers taking a prenatal nutritional supplement.

Your partner's doctor may want to perform a physical exam that will measure her vital signs such as her blood pressure, weight, and height. Included in the physical exam would be a breast exam and pap smear, unless she has done one recently. Blood and urine tests may also be performed to confirm the pregnancy and check for things such as anemia, urinary tract infection, Rh factor, blood type, and sexually transmitted infections, to name a few. The health practitioner who is checking the health of the mother is doing so to determine her general health and to check if there may be any precautions that need to be taken.

What You Should Do

Prepare for morning sickness by having small snacks ready for your partner to munch on. Do not allow her to go long periods without eating; meal portions should be snack-sized. Try to stay away from food that has complex flavors or smells, as these may aggravate the nausea. Stick to plain foods that are high in carbohydrates, like plain toast, pasta, biscuits, crackers, and anything with ginger in it. This will help in reducing nausea and vomiting.

Make sure your partner is well hydrated, and offer her water, sparkling water, and fruit juice often. If the morning sickness is so bad that your partner is throwing up everything, make sure she seeks medical attention, as she may have hyperemesis gravidarum, an extreme type of morning sickness where a woman vomits more than four times a day. A woman with hyperemesis gravidarum may be at risk of dehydration, dizziness, and losing a large amount of weight.

Introduce a routine where you take an early morning or late evening walk with your partner. This will give you time to listen to your partner and allow them time to rant about all the changes they are feeling. Walks are a form of exercise that your partner can take part in all the way until her third trimester. Swimming and yoga are also types of exercises that your pregnant partner can do with you that are safe for them to do in their pregnant state. To combat her constipation, include fruit, vegetables, lentils, brown rice, or any other insoluble fiber to her diet.

Be patient as your partner experiences these extreme changes to their body and hormones. It can get frustrating for a pregnant woman who is experiencing the pregnancy symptoms for the first time. Accompany your partner to all her prenatal doctor's appointments if you can, so that she doesn't feel alone. Bad news may come at any time; it is important you show that you support her by being present as she goes through every stage. Milestones should be celebrated, and you should also be present for all the good stuff as well. Once something has passed, you do not get that time back.

What You Should Not Do

Do not force your partner to eat things that make them feel worse. It is understandable that you may be worried about the overall health of your partner, and seeing how much they are vomiting and how little they are eating may be alarming to you. If they are drinking little sips and eating a few bites here and there, it will be enough to get them through. Your partner is going through so many different changes, so take each day as it comes and listen. I made a lot of mistakes listening to other females in my life when it came to pregnancy, instead of listening to my wife.

Had I just taken the time to listen to what she was feeling and what she felt like she needed, I would not have gotten myself and her so frustrated. It is all about patience, trial, and error. Your partner may be able to stomach crackers today and instantly vomit them tomorrow. They may be repulsed by the smell of cinnamon this week and crave it the next week. Your job is to remain flexible and go with the flow. Do not forget to reassure her that she is glowing and that whatever physical changes she is going through suit her and make her more beautiful than she already is.

In the last weeks of the first trimester, your baby will be finishing off the development of certain systems in their body. During this stage, your partner may also develop a baby bump, which will make this even more real for the both of you. The pregnancy symptoms will rage on and you will have to continue to be the reassuring support system you have become for your partner. The next chapter will walk you through all these exciting changes. Just keep reading, Dad!

Chapter 3
First Trimester (9–13 weeks)

You're almost at the end of the beginning. It can be hard for a couple to adjust to the pregnancy between the ninth and thirteenth week because, during this time, symptoms like morning sickness, fatigue, and heartburn are often at their peak. Your partner is probably feeling very uncomfortable during this time. In spite of these symptoms, the first trimester often flies by, and once your partner reaches 13 weeks, the risk for miscarriage significantly drops. It doesn't necessarily mean she's out of danger, but you can breathe a little easier.

There are also some considerations to make in terms of which food and activities that you can partake in with your partner while they are pregnant. Keeping both your partner and the baby safe during pregnancy will help increase the chances that the pregnancy will be a viable one. Keeping these considerations in mind may help you take better care of your pregnant partner and help her avoid danger.

Getting Past the Danger Zone

Let's Talk About Sex

In order to get close to your partner, you likely have sex often. Sex is another way you can get closer to your partner to show them how passionate you feel about them. Sex is also how you got her pregnant. Sex is a wonderful experience that should happen between two consenting adults. But what if one of them is pregnant: Can you still have sex? The question of sex during pregnancy is one that brings hesitation to a lot of couples. You may be hesitant to make love to your partner because you may worry that you are hurting her or the baby. If she's been having a miserable time due to her symptoms, this may also add to your hesitancy.

Unless there are concerns from your partner's doctor, sex during pregnancy is allowed and encouraged for the duration of the pregnancy. Sex will add intimacy to your relationship and give your partner a sense of comfort, as long as she is up to it. There is no danger to your baby when you have sex with your partner when is she is pregnant. Your penis cannot reach your partner's uterus while your baby is safely growing within it. Moreover, the cervix provides even more protection to ensure that nothing enters the uterus. "As long as your partner does not have unexpected vaginal bleeding, a history of preterm labor or cervical insufficiency, or a concerning complication, sex during pregnancy is generally considered safe" (Pevzner, 2021g).

There are many benefits that you and your partner can benefit from during pregnancy. The bond you share can be deepened by having regular sexual relations with your partner while they are pregnant. Due to the increased blood flow to the genitals, a woman may experience more intense and powerful orgasms that last for longer. Sex is a physical activity and therefore it burns calories; the more sex you and your partner have, the more calories you burn, which adds to your overall fitness. There have been studies to suggest that sex releases an antibody that successfully fights bacteria that bring colds and other infections to the body.

Overall, you want to keep your partner happy and satisfied. Sex will allow you to do so, as orgasms increase happiness. When your pregnant partner orgasms, their body will release endorphins that will give them "feel-good vibes". These endorphins not only make the mom-to-be happy, they also make the baby feel happy, too. You may find your partner more attractive due to the changes in her body (increased breast size, wider hips, glowing skin) and she may have an increased sex drive due to the increased blood flow to her reproductive organs. All these things make it a perfect recipe for you and your partner to grow closer in intimacy while she is growing a miracle in her body.

My wife started to develop some insecurities as her pregnancy developed. One of the ways I got to show her how much I appreciate her and to express how attractive I found her in her pregnant state was to make love to her. I didn't think she would be up to it half of the time because of how sick she was, but she would initiate sex a majority of the time. Your journey may be different depending on your circumstances and how pregnancy affects your partner, but always remember that sex is on the table.

Do Not Eat This, Do Not Drink That

There are a lot of myths and old wives' tales about what should be ingested by a pregnant woman. The truth is she can eat anything she wants, aside from a handful of foods that may be harmful to her and the growing embryo. The following list of foods and beverages should be avoided or kept to a minimum in order to avoid risks such as miscarriage and developmental issues in the growing baby.

Caffeine

A lot of adults survive life through caffeine. I cannot start my day as a father of three without caffeine; the same goes for my partner. Although caffeine is not a big no-no during pregnancy, the American College of Obstetricians and Gynecologists (ACOG) advises pregnant women to limit their intake of caffeine to not more than 200 mg, which is around 3.5 oz. The reason caffeine should be limited is that it passes through to the placenta quite easily, but the baby does not yet have the enzyme needed to break it down. This means that the caffeine levels can build up in the placenta causing restricted fetal growth, which increases the chances of low birth weight. This then increases the risk of infant death and a higher chance of developing chronic disease when the baby reaches adulthood.

Alcohol

This is a tricky one, because there's no level of alcohol that has been proven safe during pregnancy. If you don't know what levels are safe to take, it's better to avoid alcohol entirely. Your partner indulging in alcohol while she is pregnant is dangerous, because it increases the risk of giving birth to a stillborn baby or her miscarrying the pregnancy. Drinking while pregnant also increases the chance of the baby contracting fetal alcohol syndrome, which may cause heart defects, facial deformity, and some intellectual disabilities. If you want to give the baby the best start that they can get in life, allowing your partner to indulge in alcohol while pregnant is jeopardizing this chance at a good start.

High-Mercury Fish

Mercury is an element that is highly toxic if you are exposed to it in high amounts. It may affect your kidneys, immune system, and nervous system. It is a pollutant in water and therefore, it can be found in certain fish. High-mercury fish to avoid include swordfish, shark, tuna, king mackerel, and marlin. Not all fish will be high in mercury; you need to be vigilant about which fish your partner consumes. Low-mercury fish include salmon, tilapia, trout, cod, and anchovies. To avoid the complications that mercury may have on your developing baby, it is best that mom-to-be does not ingest high-mercury fish at all.

Shellfish and Raw Fish

This may be a difficult one to adjust to if you and your partner regularly eat sushi. Raw fish and raw shellfish can be the cause of a variety of viral, parasitic, or bacterial infections such as listeria, salmonella, and norovirus. Depending on the infection, it may only affect you, or it may be passed onto your unborn baby and may cause various dire consequences. These infections can cause premature delivery, stillbirth, miscarriage, and other health issues; therefore, it is not worth it.

Raw Eggs

Salmonella bacteria may be found in raw eggs. If you and your partner eat eggs that are not cooked but contain this salmonella bacteria, then you may experience nausea, vomiting, fever, stomach cramps, as well as diarrhea. Although it is rare, it is possible that a salmonella infection will result in uterine cramps that lead to stillbirth or premature birth. Various foods contain raw eggs, such as hollandaise sauce, homemade salad dressings and mayonnaise, lightly scrambled eggs, and poached eggs. If a product is made with pasteurized raw eggs, then it is safer to consume, but you should read the label thoroughly before allowing your partner to ingest the product. To be safe, simply cook your eggs until there are no signs of runny yolk.

Raw/Undercooked Meat

The same way raw fish is affected by bacteria when it is undercooked or raw, meat also contains several types of bacteria and parasites that could increase the risk of infection in a pregnant woman. Infections that result in E. coli, salmonella, listeria, and toxoplasma can be contracted when a pregnant woman eats undercooked or raw meat. The only meat you should serve your pregnant partner should be cooked through, and you should avoid giving her processed meat unless you have cooked it through as well. Processed meat can contract bacteria when it's being processed or during storage.

Organ Meats

Organ meat is a delicious source of a variety of nutrients that include vitamin A, zinc, iron, and vitamin B12. However, it is advised that a pregnant woman avoids too much vitamin A, as it may lead to miscarriage and congenital malformations. You can still serve your partner organ meat as long as you keep its consumption to a few ounces in a week. This applies to vitamin A supplements as well: Keep them at a minimum.

Raw Sprouts

Sprouts are often included in meals either as a garnish or as a tasty addition to salads. Mung bean sprouts, alfalfa, radish, and clover sprouts are some of the more popular sprouts that are commonly ingested. Unfortunately, due to the humid environment in which sprouts usually begin to grow, they are often riddled with bacteria, such as salmonella. These bacteria are nearly impossible to wash off; therefore, a pregnant woman should not consume raw sprouts at all. If she insists on having sprouts, then you should cook them well before she eats them to kill off any bacteria.

Unwashed Fruit and Vegetables

Fruit and vegetables pass through many hands and chemicals before they land in your fridge or on your table. There are various types of bacteria that could be acquired either through the soil the produce was growing in or via their handling. These bacteria may lead to infection such as E. coli, salmonella, listeria, and toxoplasma. If a baby contracted toxoplasma while they were in the womb and is born with no symptoms, they may develop them later in life, such as blindness or intellectual disability. Always wash fruit and vegetables thoroughly with running water before eating with your partner. You can also cook or peel produce to reduce the risk of infection.

Unpasteurized Dairy Products

Soft, unpasteurized cheese and raw milk can also contain harmful bacteria that can lead to infection for both mom and baby. In terms of bacteria, the usual suspects are involved, including E. coli, listeria, salmonella, and campylobacter. Basically, anything unpasteurized is bad, and that also includes fruit juice. Pasteurization is important because it serves as the most effective method of killing harmful bacteria without destroying any of the nutrition in the milk or juice. Do not serve your pregnant partner anything that is unpasteurized, or any soft cheese.

What's Happening to Baby

At nine weeks the baby is around one inch long and their physical features are becoming more human by the day, with the fingers and toes becoming more defined and the earlobes and tip of the nose becoming more distinguishable. The liver, pancreas, and bile ducts are forming this week, but more notable is that the baby is now wiggling about and these movements can be seen on the ultrasound. At 10 weeks, this is your baby's final week as an embryo. Their major organs have begun to form, their nose, eyes, and mouth are even more defined, and their tooth buds are taking shape. Outer ears are recognizable and the eyelids are beginning to close.

At 11 weeks, your baby is no longer an embryo, but is now a fetus. Your baby is now around 2 inches long; all organs began development in the embryo stage and will now mature in the fetal stage. The fetus is moving its arms and legs around, although those movements cannot yet be felt. Taste buds are developing, and the eyelids will fuse shut. The webbing between fingers and toes has disappeared and the fetus has more defined limbs. When your baby reaches 13 weeks, they will look like a tiny, fully formed human measuring around 2.5 inches. Your baby's skeleton is hardening and their fingernails are forming.

Your baby's skin is still see-through and delicate. The vocal cords are forming and the liver has just begun generating red blood cells. Another exciting thing that is happening at 12 weeks is that hormones are being secreted by the fetus's pituitary gland. By the end of this week, the baby's intestines will make their way into their abdomen, where there is finally enough room to accommodate them. The placenta is also now fully functional and can take over hormone production that is meant to sustain the pregnancy. At 13 weeks your baby is now producing urine and releasing it into the amniotic fluid, where they swallow it again. They are developing hair follicles as well as fingerprints. The placenta continues to provide the baby with oxygen as well as nutrients, while filtering out its waste produce. The fetus is now 3 inches long.

What's Happening to Mom

Your partner is experiencing heightened symptoms during the ninth week and she may also experience itchy breasts, heartburn, and extreme mood swings. Progesterone and other hormone fluctuations are responsible for a majority of these symptoms. By 10 weeks, your partner will still probably be struggling with fatigue, nausea, frequent urination, and constipation. Due to the frequent urination, your partner may experience disturbances in her sleep schedule; she may also experience weird dreams. Breaks in sleep will also exacerbate her fatigue. Your partner may also experience more headaches.

Chorionic villus sampling (CVS) may be offered to couples between 10 and 12 weeks who are 35 or older, have a child who has a genetic disorder, or have a history of genetic disorders. This testing is done in order to detect chromosomal abnormalities. At 11 weeks your partner's belly may begin to show, especially if this is not her first pregnancy or if she's carrying multiples. This may also be a good time for you and your partner to have a discussion with both your supervisors about her pregnancy and maternity and paternity leave.

By 12 weeks, your partner's uterus is starting to grow too big and will spill out of her pelvis. Levels of hCG may begin to level off during this time and this will ease the nausea and vomiting. Due to the uterus moving out of the pelvis, the frequent urination might be eased as well. By the time 13 weeks rolls around, your partner will be in her last week of the first trimester. She may start to develop some stretch marks and notice clear or white vaginal discharge, which is normal during pregnancy. This discharge is called leukorrhea. Your partner's appetite may return as her nausea decreases, and it is important to always offer her healthy food choices so that she can maintain her health and that of the baby.

What You Should Do

You can begin a video or picture journal that documents the growth of your partner's expanding abdomen. There are a million ideas online on how you can document your partner's pregnancy journey. It is always a tear-jerking journey down memory lane that you can share with your baby when they are grown up. Anything you can save during the pregnancy journey can be put in a memory box as keepsakes.

Encourage your partner to take naps during the day to alleviate their fatigue. Designate nap times where your partner can take a time out and rest. These periodic rest periods may help her to feel more energized, which will also assist in stabilizing her moods. Find your partner stretchy pants with an elastic waistline to accommodate her growing abdomen. You can offer to moisturize your partner's abdomen with some tissue oil in order to care for her skin, but it is important to note that stretch marks are normal and they will often fade over time after the baby is born.

What You Should Not Do

Do not reveal news of the pregnancy or details about your partner's health condition or struggles unless you have the permission of your partner. It is your journey too, but it is her body. I made the mistake of oversharing how constipated my wife was, and she did not appreciate that at all. Only share what you and your partner are comfortable sharing. Make sure you have her express consent to share certain details to avoid misunderstandings.

Do not comment on how your partner has changed or what they do not do anymore since they became pregnant. Pregnancy is a difficult adjustment for your partner and there are also some self-esteem issues they may experience. Rapid weight gain, larger breasts, and wider hips may result in your partner experiencing insecurities tied to her self-image; she may also experience bloating that makes her look further along than she is in the pregnancy. Do not make remarks about your partner's body or changes in her behavior.

If the pregnancy reaches 13 weeks, then congratulations, as it means that the risk of a miscarriage is a greatly reduced and you are now headed into the second trimester. At this point, you will now be facing many great milestones, such as finding out the sex of the baby as well as feeling the baby move for the first time. You will also have a front row seat as your partner's abdomen expands in direct proportion to the growth of your baby. The closer you get to the due date, the more excited you will become. The next chapter will take you through the first few weeks of the second trimester and what that will look like for the mom-to-be and the baby. I have taken you this far, I am not about to leave you hanging!

Chapter 4
Second Trimester (14–17 weeks)

Now that your partner has reached the second trimester, she is a third of the way there. The following weeks may feel a lot easier and more comfortable for the mom-to-be as her hormones become more stable. Due to the stabilization of the pregnancy hormones, she may also regain her energy. The biggest milestone that will bring some relief to couples at this stage is not worrying so much about early pregnancy loss. Unfortunately, not all couples will breathe a sigh of relief until they have their baby safely within their arms, but getting to the second trimester is a major step in the right direction.

Get Ready for Another Hormonal Shift

You may have been waiting for the second trimester to kick in so that your partner does not have to suffer morning sickness and all of the other symptoms she may have been experiencing. Fortunately, for most women, the second trimester does come with the advantage of waning pregnancy symptoms. This does not mean that other changes won't happen. On the contrary, more changes are on the way. Think of your partner as an unpredictable cauldron of hormones that can react in different ways on different days. It is said that preparation is the mother of success, and I want to keep you prepared for what may come in the second trimester.

Your partner may begin to experience a change in their joints and muscles, which may feel strange to them. Relaxin is a hormone that assists in the relaxation of muscles in the pelvis (including the uterus and cervix) that also assists in the growth of the placenta. This hormone is great if you are partaking in activities such as prenatal yoga, but it can prove detrimental and lead to aches and pains in the joints and ligaments. Due to the relaxation of these muscles, it can lead it to a higher risk of injuries. I began to really believe this when my wife explained to me that it felt as if something was clicking every time she walked. Sometimes she would have to rest for some time to ease the pain, but it disappeared after she gave birth.

Another change that may happen in the second semester, due to hormone changes, is the mask of pregnancy (melasma). Although the hormones are stabilized, their levels are still increasing. As estrogen and progesterone increase, it may cause your partner's melanocytes cells to produce more melanin, and melanin is what is responsible for your skin color. This may cause your partner to develop gray or brown patches on their face. Not only that, but you may notice that their nipples become darker and their moles are more pronounced. A line that divides their belly, referred to as the linea nigra, appears out of nowhere and will become dark and pronounced. Fortunately, none of these changes to your partner's skin are permanent and will disappear not too long after birth.

Cortisol is a hormone that is responsible for the regulation of multiple processes in the human body, which also include your metabolism and immune response. During pregnancy, cortisol increases. It may be known as a stress hormone, but it also controls and regulates blood sugar levels. When levels of cortisol increase, it also creates unwanted pregnancy symptoms such as stretch marks, redness in the face, as well as blood pressure problems. In order to aid the growth of the fetus, human placental lactogen (HPL) is released by the placenta. HPL may also cause gestational diabetes, which can cause the baby to grow too big.

What's Happening to Baby

At 14 weeks, your baby is around 3.5 inches long and they are about 3 oz in weight; the fetus is around the size of a lemon. An exciting development is that your baby is now able to make different facial expressions; they can squint, frown, and pucker their lips. The reason your baby can now grimace and pull various other faces is because of their developing brain impulses. Fine hairs (lanugo) are beginning to cover your baby's entire body. As your baby's liver produces bile, their kidneys continue to produce urine as a way to prepare the baby for the outside world.

When the baby reaches 15 weeks, they will be around the size of an apple or an orange, and they are now constantly moving about. The skin is becoming less translucent and hair is growing rapidly all over the body, including the eyebrows. Development of the skeleton is also in full swing. At 16 weeks the fetus is now measured up from their crown, which is their head, to their rump, which is in their bottom. At this stage they were about 4.5 inches long and around 3.5 oz, which is around the size of an avocado.

Your baby at 16 weeks has better-functioning urinary and circulatory systems. Their head is straightening out and appearing less angled forward; the eyes and ears are positioned where they will sit permanently. If your baby is a girl then all of her eggs are slowly developing within her ovaries. When your baby reaches 17 weeks, more developments are in tow. "Around 5 inches in length and weighing in at about 4 to 5 ounces, your baby is now bulking up. Their skeleton, which has been comprised primarily of soft cartilage, is now transitioning into solid bone" (Schaeffer, 2017b). Your baby is growing more fat, as they will need it in order to regulate their body temperature.

Your baby can now make sucking motions with their mouth and, although their sucking is not coordinated with their swallowing, this will mature closer to the end of the pregnancy. The umbilical cord and placenta are in rapid development and doing their best to provide for your baby. The umbilical cord is expanding in size and length in order to meet your baby's growing needs. The placenta is also expanding in order to provide better circulation of nutrients and oxygen.

What's Happening to Mom

During the 14th week of pregnancy, the nausea may still linger, but should be more bearable or completely gone. If not, your partner may be one of the women who is suffering from hyperemesis gravidarum. The easing of the nausea and vomiting may help the mom-to-be regain her sex-drive and want to possibly reignite the intimacy in the relationship; she will still be experiencing emotional shifts; therefore, more changes are afoot. At 15 weeks pregnant your partner may be experiencing body aches, continued weight gain, carpal tunnel syndrome in the hands and feet, as well as changes in her skin around the nipple area.

When your partner reaches 16 weeks of the pregnancy, they may become a little forgetful or experience what is termed as "pregnancy brain." She may also have trouble concentrating. The symptoms that she experiences this week may not be new ones, but she may start to look like she has a pregnancy glow due to increased blood flow and hormones that may make her skin shinier and oilier. The most exciting thing that happens this week is that your partner may get to feel your baby moving around in her uterus. You might not get to feel the baby moving for a few more weeks though, so be patient.

As your baby grows, there is limited space in your partner's abdomen for her organs. Due to this, she may develop gastrointestinal issues such as heartburn and indigestion. This will happen around 17 weeks; your partner will perhaps experience some nausea or heartburn that may rise to her throat and make her more uncomfortable. Heartburn can feel a lot like you are dying, but it is generally not harmful. In order for your partner to avoid heartburn, they should not eat large portions in one sitting. Small snack-sized meals are what is recommended and what you should serve her. If the heartburn is not getting better and causing a lot of discomfort, then your partner's doctor may be able to offer her antacids that are safe for the baby.

The gastrointestinal issues don't stop at heartburn and indigestion; they also include gas and constipation. These are symptoms that are often present in early pregnancy, but they can get worse as the pregnancy goes on. In order to counter constipation and gas, your partner simply needs to make lifestyle changes so that she can reduce discomfort. There isn't much you or your partner can do about the hormonal changes that caused the gas and constipation, but you can make sure your partner increases her water intake and that she is eating more fiber.

Your partner may also begin to complain about random shooting pains from either one of her legs. This can happen because of the sciatic nerve, which is the largest nerve in the human body. Although it is not quite known why pregnant women experience sciatic nerve pain, it is suspected that due to the growing uterus and the pressure it puts on the nerve, it results in pregnant women feeling intermittent pain in the lower back or hip that radiates down to their legs. The best way to treat sciatic nerve pain is to engage in low impact exercises such as swimming in order to relieve discomfort. Your partner may also lie on the side that isn't experiencing the pain with a pillow between her knees and ankles and remain in that position until the pain subsides.

Another new symptom that your partner may start to experience is nasal congestion. "It affects about 39% of pregnant people, with most cases striking between week 13 and week 21" (Pevzner, 2021h). The exact cause of why pregnant women get nasal congestion is unknown. It is suspected that a sudden increase of hormones and blood volume encourages mucus glands to overproduce, leading to nasal congestion as well as constant sneezing. Your partner may relieve nasal congestion by using saline drops or a spray, using a humidifier in the home, elevating her head when sleeping, and avoiding fumes, dust, pollen, and cigarette smoke. If none of these work for her she can approach her doctor, as nasal congestion may be indicative of other illnesses.

What You Should Do

Your partner may have their appetite back at this stage; therefore, it is important to have healthy meal options for the rest of her pregnancy.

Your partner does not have to "eat for two," but she will need to add more calories to her diet in order to make sure she is eating enough to be healthy and to support the growing baby. According to the American Pregnancy Association, 300 additional calories should be added to a pregnant woman's diet during the second trimester (Silver, 2017). Those additional calories could come from food like fruits, vegetables, low-fat dairy, lean meats, and whole grains.

Due to the many changes your partner is going through physically, it may be difficult for her to get comfortable when it is time to sleep. You can get her some pregnancy pillows that she can use to make herself more comfortable when it is bedtime. Try to get as many pillows and cushions she may need to get comfortable on the couch, in the car, at work, and in the bed. As her body changes, there will be different positions that she may be comfortable in, and pillows help to support her back, legs, and hips while she is trying to get comfortable.

A good idea would be to book your partner a prenatal massage to ease the new aches and pains she is developing as her body is changing. It is always important to notify anybody who is giving a massage that your partner is pregnant so that they take necessary precautions. Your partner will feel appreciated and pampered, and it will give her a chance to really relax. Start thinking about and discussing with your partner if you want to find out the sex of the baby, as that may come up anytime now. You will be able to find out the sex of the baby any time from 16 weeks. Gender is a big deal; start thinking about it if you want to know. You may also want to consider brainstorming baby names.

What You Should Not Do

Just because your partner is now in the second trimester does not mean you are fully out of the danger zone. Pregnancy is very unpredictable and anything can happen at any time. Do not to brush it off if your partner experiences the following symptoms:

- vaginal bleeding or spotting
- signs of labor

- shortness of breath or difficulty breathing
- severe abdominal cramping

If your partner experiences any of these symptoms, you should take her to the emergency room immediately or contact her doctor.

The second trimester is often referred to as "honeymoon pregnancy" due to the fact that morning sickness might have eased, but your partner is still experiencing an array of pregnancy symptoms; therefore, you should still employ a sense of empathy and patience when it comes to your partner. Her body is still changing and her hormones are still raging. Now that she can see her belly, her anxiety about losing the baby might increase instead of decrease. Do your best to check in with her mental health to see if she is coping with all the changes that are going on with the baby and her body. Do not neglect her mental and emotional well-being.

The next chapter is an exciting one! Speaking about gender and whether or not you want to know before the baby is born is a vital part of your pregnancy journey. In the next chapter we will explore why people want to know the gender of their baby before it is born and how that is done. There are a lot of myths out there about gender prediction, from the shape of the belly and how it's sitting, to using the lunar calendar. It is also exciting for parents to imagine themselves as a mother and father to a baby girl or a baby boy. Gender makes the pregnancy experience much more real. If you stick around, I will walk you through it. Are you ready?

Chapter 5
Second Trimester (18–22 weeks)

During this phase of the pregnancy, you and your partner are basically halfway through the pregnancy. There is no doubt that you have been tested quite a few times mentally and emotionally. Being a support system for your pregnant partner is not easy at times, so I would like to commend you for being there and getting through it. Pregnancy is not only about your partner; pregnancy involves you too. You planted the seed and she's doing the growing. You're equally important during the journey, just like you'll be equally important during your child's life. We all have a role to play.

I remember how much I struggled with feeling helpless. When my wife was sick and throwing up, all I could do was rub her back, hold her hair, and bring her sparkling water afterward. I couldn't feel her aches and pains and I couldn't take her discomfort away. When I expressed how detached I felt, she told me that we were in this together, but we played different roles and would inevitably walk different paths during the pregnancy. She told me her job was to carry and birth the baby, and my job was to be there and support her. If you're supporting your partner in every way you can, you are doing a good job.

This is an exciting time as your partner may be looking more beautiful than ever with her radiant skin and cute baby bump, but I'm not talking about how beautiful she is. I'm talking about gender. The time has come for you to finally decide if you want to know or if you're keeping it a surprise. Some people like to remain old-school and find out the gender when the baby is born. Regardless of what you or your partner chooses, the ball is in your court as long as you make the decision together.

Let's Talk Gender

From the moment you find out that your partner is expecting, you are likely to fantasize about the sex of the baby. It's so rewarding to wonder and explore the possibilities about having a little boy or a little girl. Not only will you and your partner be curious about the sex of the baby, your friends, colleagues, family members, and possibly even strangers may stop and ask if you know the sex of the baby. A follow-up question if you answer no would be if you intend to find out the sex of the baby.

There are so many myths surrounding how to predict the sex of the baby, and many couples partake in trying to guess or predict the sex before it is confirmed by an ultrasound. "While some 'theories' sound scientific and may even appear to be legitimate, most lack any hard evidence... These 'tips and tricks' are, at most, a source of entertainment (as long as they're safe for the parent and fetus)" (Gurevich, 2021).

Why You Should Find Out the Sex of the Baby

There are many good reasons why parents should want to know what the sex of the baby is before the baby is born. Waiting nine months to find out specific details about your baby may be too much for some parents to handle. Some couples cannot live with that big of a curiosity for that long. It will depend on you and your partner and your personality types if you can thrive under the suspense of waiting. If you are not able to wait that long, then it's okay to find out what the sex of your baby is.

When you know such a big detail about your baby before the birth, it can create an early bond between you and your baby. When you know that your baby is a little girl, you can imagine all the tea parties you might have or envision what kind of teenager she may be; your mind can take you as far as her wedding day, when you'll have the opportunity to walk her down the aisle. If it's a little boy, you can envision having those one-on-one moments that you may have had with your own father. Or, if your father was not in your life, it's exciting to think of all of the new traditions you can start with your son.

Knowing the sex of your baby allows you to brainstorm all of the possible names that you could give them. Your partner may want to name your baby after her grandmother on her mother's side, or you may want to give the child a family name that has been passed down for generations. Maybe one of you wants to name the child Pear. Naming your baby is a big deal, and when you find out the sex early on, you and your partner will have ample time to debate and discuss your baby's name long before they are born.

In order to prepare for the arrival of the baby, it is helpful to know what the sex of the baby is in order to plan gender specific parties or decide on colors for the nursery. This will also give you the opportunity to arrange a gender reveal party or register at baby shops knowing what colors you want your friends and family to buy for the baby. Lastly, knowing the sex of your baby can be beneficial in terms of prenatal monitoring of certain congenital diseases that affect one gender more than the other.

Why You Should Wait to Find Out the Sex of the Baby

Not every couple will decide to find out the sex of the baby. Some couples actually prefer the surprise of finding out the sex of the child when they are born. There are various reasons why parents of an unborn child may decide to wait and opt out of finding out the baby's sex. Some people genuinely would love to be surprised at birth. For them, the need to be surprised overpowers the curiosity to find out before the baby is born. It may sound old-fashioned, but there are some people who go through the pregnancy without knowing the sex of the child.

Another reason why couples may opt to wait rather than find out the sex of the baby is to avoid gender disappointment. As a parent, you may have a strong preference as to which sex you would prefer. Some parents may decide to find out the sex before the baby is born so that they can work through their disappointment. Others may decide to find out at birth because the joy of the birth will cancel out their disappointment. Gender disappointment is a phenomenon that you may not expect to feel until it happens to you.

There are some cultures around the world that believe that it is bringing bad luck in the family if the pregnant couple finds out the sex before birth. Some religions even go as far as theorizing that finding out the sex before birth goes against God's plan as he intended you to know the sex of the child at the birth of that child. In some families it is a tradition to wait for the baby to be born and find out then what the sex of the baby is. And then there are those couples that are not interested in gender stereotypes, so it doesn't matter to them what the sex of the baby is, because they have chosen gender-neutral items for their nursery and neutral-colored clothes.

Whatever you decide for your family is neither right nor wrong. Speak with your partner candidly and express yourself clearly while also giving her the opportunity to express herself as well. These are topics that you should take seriously, because once you have decided to know, you can never erase the moment. There are also couples that find out the sex of the baby but decide to keep it to themselves; their friends and family will only find out when that baby is born. What matters is that you and your partner are on the same page and no one is forcing their will upon the other.

Scientific Methods That Predict Sex

Ultrasound

Your partner's healthcare provider may decide to perform an ultrasound between 18 and 22 weeks in order to determine the sex of the baby. During this appointment, the ultrasound is done in order to assess the development of the baby and if their organs are developing correctly. The ultrasound technician is able to see your baby's genitals and be correct about the sex with almost 100% accuracy. In the case of a female child, the technician knows to look for the hamburger sign that is indicative of female genitalia. With a male child, the penis may be visible. The technician can either announce the sex or write it on a piece of paper.

Chorionic Villus Sampling (CVS)

This test is not performed for sex prediction only, but it is also usually requested to assess for chromosomal abnormalities. With CVS, tissue that is taken from the placenta is what the tests will be performed on; unfortunately, this kind of testing is risky and there is a small possibility that the pregnant woman may develop an infection or miscarry the fetus. When this type of test is being carried out, the parents of the baby can request sex prediction as well.

Amniocentesis

Similar to the CVS test, amniocentesis comes with its risks. It is performed by inserting a needle into the amniotic sac through the abdomen; the person performing this test will be guided by an ultrasound as the needle collects amniotic fluid. The amino test is done in such a way that it won't harm the fetus. The reason why this test is usually done is to analyze genetic material present in amniotic fluid. Analyzing the amniotic fluid helps with chromosomal analysis and detection of certain genetic diseases. While this test is being administered, the parents can request for sex prediction.

Non-Invasive Prenatal Testing (NIPT)

This is a low-risk test that is primarily used to screen for congenital diseases. This is a new type of prenatal test that assesses DNA that is free-floating in the blood (cfDNA). A pregnant woman carries the cfDNA of her unborn child in the placenta. What is found in the placenta is genetically identical to what would be found in the fetus. If the Y chromosome is present in the cfDNA fragments, then the fetus is a boy. If the Y chromosome is absent, then it is assumed that the fetus is a girl.

Non-Scientific Methods That Predict Sex

There is no way to prove the accuracy of these theories, but they have often been used to try to predict the gender of the baby. Some people believe that if you are carrying a girl child, you will have more severe morning sickness. Others believe that the parents' intuition is enough to predict the sex of the baby. Under this theory, your partner's guess is likely correct because a parent "just knows". There is also the theory that the faster the heart of the fetus beats, the more likely it is a female.

There is a common theory that if a woman carries high, the baby is likely to be a boy and if she carries low, the baby is a boy. A baking soda test can apparently also predict the sex of your baby. To perform the baking soda test, mix your partner's urine with the baking soda, and if it reacts by bubbling or fizzing then your baby is male; if nothing happens, they are female. There are millions of non-scientific sex prediction tests online that you can do with your partner in order to predict the sex of the baby. There's no harm in doing these tests, but do not pin your hopes on any of them.

What's Happening to Baby

At 18 weeks, your baby is undergoing major changes with regard to their senses. They are 5.5 inches long and they weigh 7 ounces. At this stage they are roughly the size of a bell pepper. Your baby's eyes are going to pop out of their head as they develop; they can detect light and are facing forward. The ears have also popped out of the head; your baby is likely to be able to hear you now. Your baby's nervous system is in serious development too, as their nerves are now covered in myelin, which allows the nerves to communicate with one another. The sex of the baby can be discerned from this point forward via an ultrasound.

When your baby reaches 19 weeks, they will be 7 inches long and around the size of an heirloom tomato. The kidneys continue to produce urine. The baby's brain is developing its sensory parts. The hair on your baby's head is starting to grow and lanugo is covering more of the body. "On top of that is vernix caseosa, the oily substance that protects the skin while the baby is growing in the womb" (Roland, 2017b). If your baby is a girl, her uterus has formed and her ovaries contain around six million eggs. At 20 weeks your baby is 1o inches long. This is the halfway point of the pregnancy.

When your baby is 21 weeks old, they are just over the halfway mark and will be 8.5 inches from crown to heel. The baby's eyes are now able to open. The development of their fingers and toes makes their hand and foot prints more noticeable. By 22 weeks, your baby is now the size of a papaya and weighs almost 1 pound. At 7.5 inches in length, your baby now resembles a small infant. Your baby has eyelids and tiny eyebrows; they are also learning to grasp with their hands. The baby is now starting to notice the sounds in their environment (your partner's body) like the rumbles of a hungry tummy or the sound of her voice. The baby is looking more like what you'd expect one to look like.

What's Happening to Mom

When your partner reaches 18 weeks, she may experience milder symptoms and bouts of increased energy. Body aches and carpal tunnel syndrome may bother her; the latter is caused by nerves being compressed in the wrist, which results in discomfort, tingling sensations, pain, and possibly numbness in the hand and arm. Carpal tunnel syndrome usually resolves after pregnancy. Body aches come about due to the growth of the uterus and the weight it places on the pelvic bones. This will manifest backache and pain in the thighs. Massage is usually the solution, and finding time to relax. Hot or cold compresses will also help relieve the discomfort.

At 19 weeks, your partner may develop what is referred to as round ligament pain. This type of pain may be felt in the abdomen and it may travel down to your partner's groin. It happens because of the stretching of the round ligament that joins the groin to the front of the uterus. At 20 weeks, an ultrasound will be performed that will last longer than any other ultrasound. The 20-week scan is the anatomy scan. During this scan, the amniotic fluid will be measured, and the baby will be measured to ensure they are growing adequately. Your partner may also get a trans-vaginal scan to check her cervix; the sex of the baby may be revealed or confirmed at this appointment.

Once your partner is 21 weeks pregnant, additional symptoms she may experience include varicose veins and urinary tract infections. To reduce the appearance of varicose veins, keep your partner's legs elevated, make sure she maintains a healthy weight and she should not remain in one position for too long. Symptoms of a urinary tract infection include pain or burning during urination, frequent urination, fever, and chills. To treat it, your partner's doctor will prescribe antibiotics; if it is left untreated, it can cause kidney infection. At 22 weeks, the pregnancy symptoms that your partner has been experiencing will continue. Hemorrhoids may develop because of the added pressure the uterus places on the anus. Added fiber and drinking plenty of fluids will aid in the relief of hemorrhoid creation; your partner may also obtain over-the-counter hemorrhoid cream.

It also may be time for your partner to consider maternity clothes and wearing things that she feels comfortable in. Do not be surprised if she borrows some things from your closet; you want her to be comfortable no matter what she puts on. Consider saving some money in order to buy a few items to add to her wardrobe that will accommodate her changing shape. Buying a new wardrobe may uplift her spirits; there-fore, you can surprise her with this opportunity to go shopping.

What You Should Do

Try to find things that will relieve your partner's new symptoms and have an index of possible solutions so that you know what is needed when they arise. Do not be caught off guard. Stock up on the safe antacid, get the hot and cold compress. Get the massage oil and anything else you can to be able to help as best you can with your partner's preg-nancy symptoms. If you work long hours, it is time to think about reducing them, if you can, so that you can spend more time with your partner and help her around the house.

Maybe your financial situation won't allow you to take time off, and you need to take on more work to be able to provide for the baby and your partner. The best thing to do is get more organized. If there are chores you need to do around the house that you are unable to, get them done as soon as possible. Try not to make a pregnant woman nag; do not procrastinate. Make a checklist for your chores. Speaking of checklists, now is the best time to get a checklist for the baby's birth and what you will need when the baby arrives.

What You Should Not Do

The best time to start planning for the arrival of the baby is from 18–20 weeks. Your partner may have some things she's been thinking about in terms of the preparations; you have to put your heads together and choose a pediatrician for your child, as well as where your partner will birth the baby. I know it seems like you have time, but you do not. Your partner will be more proactive about the planning, as she may not want to be caught unprepared; adopt the same energy. A laissez-faire attitude will not cut it.

Congratulations for surpassing the halfway mark! It is quite a wonderful milestone to reach, and it should be celebrated. You and your partner are taking this pregnancy one day at a time, as you should. Each day that passes means you are one day closer to meeting your bundle of joy. In the next chapter we will be discussing what viability means for your family. So many unpredictable things can happen; you need to know your baby's chances of survival should their birth come prematurely. We are halfway there, but we still have a long way to go.

Chapter 6
Second Trimester (23–27 weeks)

As if things couldn't get more exciting, big things are happening before your baby in the coming weeks. You are arriving at a time where your baby's chances of survival are increasing. When the fetus reaches the age of viability, this is a huge sigh of relief for most moms. If a woman has suffered loss before, she tends to relax a little after the fetus has reached the age of viability. Of course, this doesn't mean the chances of loss are zero, but your baby can be resuscitated and respond positively to medical intervention if they are birthed before their EDD.

Your partner is in the middle of her pregnancy, but her belly is expanding at a fast pace. Your partner's symptoms are bound to be directly related to the way her body is changing. She's gaining weight, and her expanding abdomen is rearranging and squashing her internal organs. The uterus is putting pressure on the surrounding muscles and ligaments, resulting in discomfort for your partner. It's only going to get worse for her as her pregnancy continues. The physical limitations of pregnancy can become quite frustrating for women. Luckily, your partner has you.

Viability

"Doctors often consider fetal viability the point at which a baby can be resuscitated at delivery and can survive without significant morbidity"

(Danielsson, 2008). The age of viability for a fetus is usually 24 weeks' gestation. The earlier a fetus is born, the higher the risk it won't survive in the outside world. Viability can sometimes be viewed as an ethical dilemma, because it begs the question of how much intervention should be done to save the life of a premature baby. Some people are of the opinion that viability is dependent upon where the baby is born in the world and the quality of healthcare they have access to.

Most hospitals will intervene and attempt to save the life of a premature fetus if they are born at 24 weeks and onwards. Even if the baby's life is saved, their care is accompanied by extreme medical interventions, which may include invasive treatments such as mechanical ventilation and a long stay in the neonatal intensive care unit. In order to assist in the baby's nourishment, they may be fitted with a tube to assist in their eating and breathing. Some doctors may attempt to save the life of a fetus who is born between 22 and 23 weeks, but they usually have state-of-the-art neonatal intensive care units as well as experienced specialists on call.

The longer a fetus remains in the womb, the higher the chance of survival. A week in the womb can make a vast difference. A fetus that is born around 37 weeks will have a better chance of survival than one that is born before 28 weeks. The survival rate of the fetus is also heavily dependent upon where they are born, as some places have more advanced medical interventions than others. A premature baby born in a different country may have a higher chance of survival than one that is born in a country ravaged by war.

Factors Affecting Viability

There are various factors that may affect whether a baby survives or not if they are born prematurely, and they include:

- Weight at birth: A baby who is born with a higher weight has a better survival rate than one that is born with a low birth weight. There is a higher risk of health issues and disabilities developing if the baby is born with a low birth weight.

- Multiples: If the woman is carrying a single baby and gives birth to it prematurely, then it has a higher rate of survival than if she was carrying multiple babies.
- Complications: In instances where the premature birth came via Cesarean section or induction due to a medical condition such as preeclampsia or abruption of the placenta, then this affects the viability of the fetus.
- Sex: A female child has a higher survival rate than a male child.
- Deprived of oxygen: If, at any point during the birth of the premature fetus, breathing is restricted, such as when the cord is wrapped around its neck, this will definitely have a bearing on their viability.
- Steroids: When the pregnancy is threatened, doctors may prescribe steroids for the mother to take in order to encourage lung development. A baby who is prematurely born having received such interventions has a higher rate of survival, as their breathing will be affected positively.

Long-Term Effects of Premature Birth

The last weeks of pregnancy are vital, as this is when there is a lot of brain development. The brain is not the only part of the body that undergoes major developments toward the end of the pregnancy. This is when the fetus gains weight and the lungs finish their development as well. A prematurely born baby will likely face some long-term effects that affect them in different ways. There is no way to predict exactly what the long-term effects on each baby will be, and those effects depend on a variety of factors.

If the baby had to receive a lot of medical intervention in order to survive, then the risk is higher that they will experience long-term effects. Some common long-term issues that premature babies have include the following:

- Cerebral palsy: This is a common neurological movement disorder that may affect a baby if there is a disruption in the development of the brain (abnormal brain development), or if their brain experiences some kind of injury.

- Cognitive impairment: The intellectual development of the child may be negatively affected if they are born prematurely.
- Chronic disease: When a child is born prematurely, their risk for chronic diseases such as heart disease, epilepsy, asthma, feeding issues, infection, and sudden infant death syndrome is increased.
- Delays in development: There are certain developmental milestones that each child must reach at roughly the same time for them to be considered a child who is developing normally. When a child is born prematurely, they reach milestones later than their peers and appear to have a slower growth rate.
- Learning disabilities: Due to the fact that being born prematurely affects the brain, this means that children born prematurely have a higher risk of having learning disabilities, the severity of which is dependent on various factors.
- Vision/hearing impairments: It is common that a fetus that is born prematurely will experience issues with regard to their sight and their hearing.
- Mental health disorders: There is a direct link between children who are born prematurely and mental health issues such as depression, anxiety, and behavioral issues.

If your baby is born before 28 weeks, there is a 20%–50% chance that they will have long-term complications due to the preterm birth. Unfortunately, if your baby is born around 26 weeks, there is an 80% chance that they will have long-term brain issues or physical disabilities (Danielsson, 2008).

Prepare Yourself

From the ultrasounds, you may already expect to deliver a premature baby, or you may find yourself in an emergency situation where your partner needs to be induced. It will be beneficial for you and your partner to discuss the resuscitation methods that you are comfortable with for your child at different gestational ages. Unfortunately, you have to face this uncomfortable conversation so that you can consider all the options available and to get the necessary advice before these difficult decisions need to be made.

Consider asking the doctor at what gestational age your baby is expected to be born, if they are suspected to be oxygen-deprived, and how many follow-up doctor appointments will be needed once they are discharged. You can also ask if there will be any long-term effects at school or developmentally, and if there will be any interventions in their care; ask if there are alternatives to the interventions and if there are risks involved. It is not an easy position to be put in, and most parents don't expect to find themselves in this kind of situation. But it can happen to anybody; be prepared.

What's Happening to Baby

At 23 weeks your baby is just over 1 pound and is almost 1 foot long. If you were to compare them to a fruit, then they are around the size of a grapefruit or a big mango. The baby's weight gain will start to ramp up soon; the lungs are still in development, but they are not functional. In preparation for the outside world, the baby is practicing breathing-like actions. The little bean is in full motion within your partner's belly and they may wake them up as they kick and dance when your partner is lying down to sleep. The baby should not keep her up too long, as they sleep often in the womb.

Your baby will be around 10 inches long when they get to 24 weeks. Surfactant, which is made up of lipids and fats, is a substance that is produced by cells in the lungs. At this point in your baby's development, surfactant is being produced and will aid in stabilizing the air sacs in the lungs, which are needed to breathe normally. The eyebrows are more pronounced and the eyelashes and taste buds are developing. At 25 weeks your baby is 1.5 pounds in weight and 12 inches tall. The baby may begin to respond to your voice and move around when your voice is heard. Your partner is getting accustomed to feeling the baby move.

In the 26th week, your baby will develop their startle and hand reflexes. The lungs are fully formed, but not yet in use. The baby is able to sleep and wake on a set schedule. If the baby is a girl, her uterus and ovaries will move to where they should be in the abdomen; if the baby is a boy, the testicles will descend into the scrotum. By week 27, your baby will be the size of a cauliflower head. They are a tiny version of what they will resemble when they are born. The lungs are still maturing, as well as the nervous system.

What's Happening to Mom

When your partner reaches 23 weeks they may have a growing bump and some swelling in the feet and ankles. Pregnant women have been known to go up a shoe size while pregnant. As she gains more weight, this will lead to stretch marks appearing on her breasts, thighs, and abdomen. The amount of weight your partner gains during pregnancy is affected by genetics, the diet she eats, and lifestyle habits. Her breasts may begin to produce colostrum, which is the first milk that your baby will need soon after birth. Colostrum is a little thicker than breastmilk and it is packed with essential antibodies the baby needs for the first few days of life. If there's no colostrum, that is also fine, as it may appear soon before or after birth.

At 24 weeks, your partner may begin to experience false labor or Braxton Hicks contractions. These are practice contractions that she may feel occasionally, and they feel like the uterus is squeezing around the baby. They are harmless and painless most of the time. If there is any pain or if the Braxton Hicks are coming frequently, your partner could be in preterm labor and should be rushed to the hospital immediately. When your partner reaches 25 weeks, they are around six months pregnant and on the cusp of exiting the second trimester. Your partner may experience sleeping difficulties due to the changes in her body, therefore it is advised for her to sleep on her left side while her knees are bent and to use multiple pillows to support her.

With 26 weeks of pregnancy comes more discomfort. Breathing may become more challenging as the uterus takes up more space. If your partner is carrying multiple babies, her doctor will increase the frequency at which she is monitored to ensure her safety and that of the babies. At 27 weeks it may be time to begin tracking the baby's movements and making sure they do not fall to less than six to ten per hour. Your partner would have reached an important milestone by completing the second trimester at the end of this week. You have another reason to celebrate.

What You Should Do

It is not a nice thing to think about, but from this point forward, the baby can come at any time. If your partner should ever feel a gush of fluid, then you should get her to the emergency room as soon as possible. Be alert for any worrying symptoms that your partner may develop. Research preeclampsia and watch out for those symptoms, especially if your partner is at risk of developing it. If your doctor deems it necessary, he may recommend that your partner acquire a device that measures her blood pressure and monitor it daily. Ensure your partner is also screened for gestational diabetes, which only needs a glucose test to be diagnosed.

Now is a great time to think about prenatal childbirth classes. You and your partner need to be aware of what is needed of you during the birth of the baby, and this is a helpful way to get you prepared. These kinds of classes teach each of you what your roles are during birth and how you can support your partner during your baby's birth. You may take some things for granted and think you know your partner and how she should be supported. Consider yourself a fish out of water and be open to learning new ways to support your partner during this time. An important thing to note is that you may not know how she will react to the intense pain of childbirth; do you know how to calm her and give her reassurance when she is scared?

Make sure you spend a considerable amount of time talking to the baby. You don't have the baby within you; therefore, you have less bonding time. The bond you form with your baby begins before they are born, while they are in utero. There are so many things you can do to create a bond, such as reading to the baby, singing, or just simply talking. Many fathers struggle to bond with their infant children. Begin the bonding process while your partner is still pregnant, and it will come more naturally when the baby is born.

What You Should Not Do

Be wary when you get intimate with your partner not to be too enthusiastic about the nipples, as they may be producing colostrum already; they may even be feeling sensitive, so it's best to stay away from them for the time being. You may also have to adjust the positions that you usually make love in, in order to accommodate your partner's growing belly. Do not be selfish and impose what feels good to you on your partner. Accommodate her changing body and adjust the sex positions so that she is comfortable and enjoying herself. If you bought all those pillows I had suggested you buy in a previous chapter, this is where they come in handy.

Try to stay calm in every situation, even if you are concerned. Your partner is stressed out and constantly undergoing new changes due to her growing baby bump. Any pain she experiences from a sensation she has not become accustomed to can be scary. Keep her calm and have her doctor's number on call to get reassurance when it's needed. Do not dismiss her concerns. Pregnancy is unpredictable; anything can happen at any time. You would rather be wrong and everything be fine than for something to be wrong and not have it checked out. You, your partner, and the baby are better off safe than sorry.

It is such a wonderful thing to have completed the second trimester, as now your baby has a better chance of survival should they be born prematurely. Entering the third trimester means that your baby's birth is just around the corner. Do not underestimate how fast the weeks fly by. In the next chapter, I will discuss all the implications that come about when your partner's belly gets bigger. Her mobility is about to be affected, not only by her growing abdomen but also due to her compressed lungs. Your partner is about to look and feel very pregnant. It is time to consider yourself in her servitude, because things are getting tough and she will need all of your help.

Chapter 7
Third Trimester (28–31 weeks)

Your partner has made it to the third and final trimester, congratulations! In three months or less, you and your partner will be holding your baby in your arms. The pregnancy is also becoming more real to you, because you can see the belly and feel the baby moving. Your partner has been pregnant all along, but it is difficult to reconcile that with reality when she looks the same way she has always looked. When you witness your partner's expanding abdomen, you realize that it is the physical manifestation of her pregnancy.

The size of the belly or when it will pop is dependent on various factors, such as genetics and whether or not this is your partner's first pregnancy. There are also consequences that come with belly expansion. The belly is such a big part of the pregnancy that it is a topic that has to be discussed in order for you to develop a love and sympathy for your partner's expanding bump. Pregnancy affects people differently; belly expansion is not a uniform exercise that affects people the same way. It may pique your curiosity to monitor how your partner's abdomen is growing.

When my wife first began to show, I thought she looked so beautiful. Seeing how her body changed when she was pregnant gave me a new respect for her and her body. It is a miracle to watch how a woman's body adapts to and supports the growth of a fetus. I do not believe a man's body would ever be able to handle the intense and constant change that pregnancy brings. Your partner is doing something incredible with her body and you should be in awe of that; I know I was, and still am.

Big Belly Talk

When Will She Show?

When exactly a pregnant woman's belly will begin to show that she is growing a fetus within her is dependent on various factors. If this is her first pregnancy, then she may show anywhere between 12 and 16 weeks; if she has been pregnant before, she will show sooner, as her abdominal wall has been stretched before and is not as tight as before she had children. If a woman is carrying multiples, she will show sooner. The kind of body a woman has can affect when her pregnant belly will be noticed. Tall women, as well as those who are overweight, may not show until 20 weeks, whereas short or slim women may show sooner.

How Does It Expand

A woman's uterus is usually below her pelvic bone. In early pregnancy, the uterus is still small and the developing pregnancy will not be noticeable. As the fetus expands, the uterus also expands and grows above the pelvic bone and into the abdomen. This is when the pregnancy begins to show.

Effects of the Belly

Outie or Flat

Your partner's belly button is located right in the middle of her abdomen and it may be affected by the expansion of her belly. Sometimes a pregnant woman's belly button will pop out as the stump of the umbilical cord is pushed outward by the uterus. This won't necessarily happen to every pregnant woman; some will just have a flat belly button. Your partner may have an outie now and not have one in her next pregnancy. Pregnancy is very subjective.

Stretch Marks

Women are accustomed to having a few stretch marks, either on her thighs, lower back, or breasts. Due to the rapid development of the fetus and the weight gain that pregnant women are expected to experience, stretch marks are inevitable. The severity of the stretch marks that occur will depend on your partner's family history, how young she is, the amount of weight she gained during pregnancy, if she was overweight before she became pregnant, and if she's carrying a big baby. Stretch marks are considered to be hereditary and cannot be prevented with topical treatment. If your partner maintains a healthy diet and drinks plenty of water while also moisturizing her skin regularly, then she can reduce the appearance of stretch marks.

Shortness of Breath

The abdomen has limited space. The baby gets bigger every day, which causes the uterus to continue expanding into the abdominal cavity. As the uterus gets bigger, it is forcing all your partner's internal organs to move higher; all her internal organs end up squashed in the rib cage. This means that there is less room for her lungs to expand. For that, the rib cage will also change shape during pregnancy, which hinders your partner from being able to take deep breaths. This is why pregnant women get winded easily if they partake in simple physical activity.

Back Pain

Your partner's posture is bound to change as her pregnancy progresses. A woman's center of gravity is shifted as her belly expands and protrudes outward. In order to correct this shift, a woman's lower back muscles have to put in more effort, which causes back pain. Normally, the abdominal muscles maintain a healthy balance with the back muscles to keep a person's center of gravity where it should be. During pregnancy, abdominal muscles are stretched and are unable to adequately support the back muscles. The larger your partner's belly, the more she will be affected by back pain. Comfortable shoes that give support to the arch of the foot will minimize lower back pain. A woman who is pregnant should avoid high heels.

Rapid Expansion

A pregnant woman's belly expands at a steady yet slow pace. If her belly suddenly expands at a rate that is unexpected, it could be influenced by a number of factors. If the expected due date is calculated incorrectly based on irregular periods, and without an ultrasound, it may seem like your bump is developing at a much faster rate than other women at the same gestation. If a woman gained too much weight during her pregnancy or was overweight before she got pregnant, their belly may look to be larger earlier.

When a woman is carrying twins, triplets, or more babies, then her pregnancy belly will be much larger than a woman who is carrying one baby. Sometimes the reason why a pregnant woman's abdomen seems larger than it should be is because of the changes that occur in the gastrointestinal tract. Bloating and gas are a common occurrence that a pregnant woman has to put up with. Unfortunately, these gastrointestinal issues can also cause the belly to expand rapidly.

Concerning Causes of Belly Expansion

There are a number of concerning causes behind a rapidly expanding abdomen that may need to be monitored in order to keep both mom and baby safe. A woman who is caring for a fetus that measures larger than average may have to be monitored. Accommodations as to how she will deliver that baby will need to be discussed as well. A molar pregnancy occurs when only placental tissue grows, because sperm fertilized an egg that was not viable. This condition is usually caught in the first trimester due to a rapidly expanding uterus.

A large ovarian tumor may be the cause of a rapidly expanding belly. They are easily spotted during routine ultrasounds. When a pregnant woman has excess amniotic fluid in the uterus, it is referred to as polyhydramnios, which may cause the belly to expand rapidly. 20% of polyhydramnios cases also involve congenital abnormalities in the fetus, yet in 70% of these cases the cause of polyhydramnios is unknown. Much like an ovarian tumor, benign fibroid tumors can cause rapid belly expansion. These fibroids can cause pain and difficulty when urinating, but are harmless.

What's Happening to Baby

At 28 weeks your baby is steadily gaining weight and is 14.5 inches long and around 2 pounds in weight. Their eyelids are partially open and may have tiny little eyelashes. The brain is developing some deep indentations and ridges, and the brain tissue present is increasing. Your baby is blinking and making an array of faces. When they sleep, they have begun to dream as well. By 29 weeks your baby will be very active. There is still enough room for them to move around and they may push on your belly often. Your baby is now almost 3 pounds and 15 inches long. The muscles and lungs are developing fast and your baby is still gaining more weight.

When your baby reaches 30 weeks they are around the size of a cucumber; they weigh 3 pounds and between 15 and 16 inches long. Your baby's eyes are still closed, but they can kind of tell what is happening around them, such as when it is dark and when it is light. At birth your baby does not have a 20/20 vision but rather 20/400 vision. This means that they can only see things that are very close to their face. Of course, as time goes on, their vision will improve. At 31 weeks your baby is roughly the size of a coconut, coming in at almost 4 pounds in weight.

With every day that passes, your baby is getting heavier and longer. Fat is settling under the skin and giving your baby that typical newborn appearance. Also contributing to these appearance changes is the fact that the lanugo (fine hair covering the baby's entire body) is gradually disappearing. The eyes are able to focus and the development of the lungs and nervous system is almost complete. Your baby has now developed reflexes such as thumb sucking, which they do frequently.

What's Happening to Mom

Your partner is now in the last trimester of her pregnancy and is able to feel a lot of the moves that the baby makes. The baby is now shifting into the correct position for delivery with their head pointing down near the cervix. Sometimes the baby moves into position a lot later than 28 weeks, and some babies never do and they remain in a breech position until birth. Your partner may feel extra pressure pushing down onto her bladder. This is the right time to start discussing what your partner may desire for the baby's delivery.

29 weeks for your partner may mean that as she is short of breath and getting winded as she performs basic activities, such as making the bed, bathing, and getting dressed. Frequent urination becomes intensified as pressure is placed on the bladder. If your partner has elevated blood pressure, progressively swelling legs, headache that won't subside accompanied by blurry/loss of vision, and she feels nauseated or is vomiting, then she may be developing preeclampsia. This is a life-threatening condition for your baby and your partner. In this instance, she needs to see a medical professional immediately.

At 30 weeks your partner may start to lose her patience and be eager to return to normal. She may be experiencing increased fatigue and finding it difficult to fall asleep. When 31 weeks roll around, your partner is now in the home stretch. Your partner is in the last quarter of her pregnancy and she has less than 10 weeks until she gives birth. Due to the pressure the expanding uterus is placing on her bladder, she may accidentally pee just a little when she sneezes or laughs too hard. This incontinence is usually resolved after pregnancy, but should it continue, your partner can strengthen her pelvic floor muscles by doing Kegel exercises frequently.

Leg cramps can bother your partner, especially at night. The chance that blood clots can develop in her legs during pregnancy increases. Inform your doctor if she develops any painful spots that are red or warm. Ensure that she has sorted everything out with her employer in regard to her maternity leave, and confirm when she leaves work for confinement and when she is expected to return. She may be experiencing leaking breasts, frequent urination, breathlessness, hemorrhoids, leg and back pain, and constipation. All these symptoms are likely to disappear once the baby is born, but they are very normal for a woman who is 31 weeks pregnant.

What You Should Do

If you haven't already, now is a great time to sign up for prenatal classes with your partner, as well as going for breastfeeding seminars and other meetings that might equip you and your partner with the necessary skills for how to cope during labor. Our parents and grandparents had to give birth with little to no knowledge except for what their parents or grandparents taught them. Men played a minimal role in all of this and it was left to the woman to deal with everything.

You are lucky, because you do not have to remain in the backseat. You are not a passenger in the birth of your child and can take an active role to make sure everything works out well. There is a lot of information that you can equip yourself with in order to give your partner and your baby the best possible chance at having a positive birth experience. Attend everything that your partner is attending, and even look for additional classes that you can join together that will prepare you for what to expect when the baby has arrived.

The nursery should be set up by now. If not, you should think about where the baby is going to sleep and what they are going to sleep in. Is your partner going to co-sleep with the baby? If the answer is affirmative, where are you going to sleep for those early days? Picture the logistics and implement them accordingly. Maybe you would like to have the baby's crib in your room for the first few weeks and then you would like to move it to the baby's room. Whatever you decide should be planned out and executed before your partner gets too tired.

What You Should Not Do

Do not wait until the last minute to choose a pediatrician for your child. Even if your child is healthy and is developing well according to the ultrasound scans, you do not know what kind of a health condition they may be born with or may develop soon after birth. Weighing your options and checking out various pediatricians in your area allows you to choose somebody that you are confident in while you are in a clear headspace. You do not want to choose a pediatrician when you are in a mental space that is charged with emotion, such as when your baby is sick and needs immediate medical attention.

Getting to this point means that you have to get all your ducks in a row so that you and your partner are prepared for the birth of your child. In this regard, you need to begin planning every little detail that you can. The plans you make may not be what happens, but a plan gives you a sense of security and makes you feel in control. Giving birth is a terrifying experience because it is unpredictable. It is also a beautiful and powerful experience, and you should enjoy every moment of it.

Going into this special moment with your partner unprepared is like relinquishing control over the events that are about to occur. If you do not have strong ideas and details about what is supposed to happen and when, these decisions will be left to medical professionals and family members. You and your partner are likely the only people that have worked at this pregnancy together every day; therefore, important decisions should not include anybody else. If it can be controlled, you and your partner should control it. What is unpredictable will happen anyway, but if you have control over something, you should wield that control unapologetically.

Your partner will be bombarded with pain, fear, and may not be in her right mind due to the extreme stress her body will be under during birth. When she is in labor, you are in control. You can tell people around her what she wants and what she doesn't want. You are her protector. Planning every detail and knowing what is supposed to happen and when gives you an idea of what you and your partner would like to happen when your baby is born and in the moments following the birth. In the next chapter, we will take you through the various plans you need to formulate in order to be adequately prepared. A planning dad is a winning dad.

Chapter 8
Third Trimester (32–35 weeks)

You are a few weeks away from meeting your baby. Your partner is likely getting quite frustrated with the physical symptoms of pregnancy, and she may be experiencing fatigue and insomnia. The baby is at the point where most of its development is complete. Now that the majority of the pregnancy has passed, it is now time to prepare for the arrival of the baby. There are so many plans to be made that you cannot leave it to the last minute.

Your partner is preoccupied with being the host of this beautiful growing baby, therefore, this is something that you can spearhead and be in control of. There are so many unpredictable factors that can affect your partner and your baby during birth or shortly thereafter; therefore, you should keep things organized and well-thought-out.

Plans, Plans, Plans

House Maintenance

Take a walk around the house and take note of all the things that need to be fixed before the baby arrives. These may not necessarily be baby-related things; they may just be things you might not be able to do when the baby arrives. Unfortunately, this is something that I overlooked when my wife was pregnant for the first time. We had some loose boards on the roof that flew off in a storm shortly after our first baby came home from the hospital. It was not something I could put off because there was rainwater leaking into the house and I had to fix it. Our new baby did not enjoy the constant hammering that lasted for over three hours. Needless to say, my wife wasn't too impressed, either.

Fix what needs to be fixed and also check if there is additional furniture that you may need. If you are getting help from either one of your mothers (either your partner's mother or your own), or any other friend or relative, you have to think about how you will accommodate them. They will need a comfortable bed and a place where they can bathe and store their luggage. Buy an extra bed if you need to, or a blow-up mattress. Make sure that you have thought about all the additional furniture needs that may arise.

Baby Shower/Gender Reveal

The baby shower is often organized by your partner's friends or family members, but you can take part in the festivities, especially now that baby showers are also attended by men. If your partner feels strongly about the baby shower attendees being all females, it doesn't mean that you can't help with the preparation. You can help in terms of the decorations, finances, and who should be on the guest list. This is a time to show your partner how much you appreciate her; ensure that whoever is organizing the shower is not stressing her about expenses or attendance.

If you and your partner opted not to reveal the sex of your baby to your families and friends, but want to do so during a gender reveal party, allow her to guide your planning, but you should do most of the heavy lifting. Find a venue and discuss and implement how the gender of the baby will be revealed; take care of logistics such as food and invitations. Your partner may be more involved in the gender reveal then she is at her baby shower, but you should be the one who implements a lot of the planning.

Hospital Bags

Have I told you yet how unpredictable pregnancy is? Well, for the millionth time, pregnancy is unpredictable. The baby can come at any time. The further along you get, the higher this chance becomes. When your partner reaches the third trimester, you need to have a bag ready in case you have to go to the hospital for the birth of the baby or any other medical emergency. Your partner may have to go to the emergency room but end up admitted into hospital until the baby is born. There will be two bags that you need to pack: one for mom and one for baby.

Mom's bag should include the following:

- comfortable clothes that have buttons (to enable easy breastfeeding)
- toiletries (face wash, nipple cream, hairbrush, toothbrush and toothpaste, shampoo, hair ties, face wipes, deodorant, etc.)
- a robe
- the birth plan
- magazines and reading material
- a long charging cord or extension cable and adapter
- towels and pillows
- a water bottle, drinks, and snacks
- postpartum recovery products

Baby's bag should include the following:

- pediatrician's information
- a few diapers and wipes
- bum cream and powder
- car seat
- an outfit to go home in
- a few long sleeve outfits, hats, and booties/socks
- baby blankets
- receiving blankets

Your bag should include the following:

- books and magazines
- a Bluetooth speaker
- blanket and pillow
- fully charged phone or camera

Childcare/Petcare

This may not be your first child, or perhaps you have pets at home that will need to be taken care of when you have gone to the hospital. Make arrangements for any of the baby's siblings and decide if they will be taken care of at home by a family member or if they are going to this caregiver's home. Decide the same thing for your pets. Will you be taking them to a shelter or leaving them with family members? These plans should be decided and set in stone before the baby arrives.

Another thing to consider is if your child will need childcare after your partner's maternity leave ends. Think about if your child is going to have a caregiver come to the home to look after them or if you will be taking your child to a daycare. Nowadays, they take children from six months old onwards. The world is more supportive of working moms; therefore, consider where you will take your child or who will come to look after them. If you have a flexible work schedule, you can also volunteer some of your time in order to stay home and care for the new baby.

Insurance

Consider making plans for how you will add your newborn child to your medical insurance as soon as they are born. You also have to consider adding the mother of your child and the child themselves to your life insurance policies as beneficiaries. You now have a responsibility to ensure that your family is okay, and that they will be supported even if something should happen to you. Consult with your insurance company on what steps you can take to ensure that your baby and partner are covered by any insurance you have.

Birth Plan

Creating a birth plan is something that is subjective and personal to you and your partner. Birth plan templates can be downloaded online. You and your partner need to consider a few factors when coming up with your birth plan, such as your newborn baby and what they need, the type of delivery your partner wants, if your partner wants pain relief, and where she wants to give birth. After going through the online templates of birth plans, you will get an appreciation of how in-depth a birth plan can be. "You need to be flexible and prepared to do things differently from your birth plan if complications arise ... or if facilities such as a birth pool aren't available" (NHS, 2020).

A birth plan is very important and can take time to formulate; therefore, this is the perfect time to go through it with your partner. Some topics will be harder to discuss and may need longer discussions to come to a decision. For example, the idea of an epidural may sound terrifying to you, but your partner may insist upon it. There will be disagreement over certain points, but if you have the time to work through those disagreements, then everything will turn out fine. Remember that your partner's opinion may carry more weight in certain topics, as she is the one who will be physically in that position.

Meal Plans

Your meal planning begins when you pack snacks for the hospital for when your partner is in labor. You also have to consider what you both will eat after the baby is born. Your partner will likely be tired from birth; she is also adjusting to caring for herself postpartum and the newborn baby. She will not have the energy to get up and cook either for herself or for you. You can prepare some casseroles or pasta dishes, which you can then freeze for later consumption.

Meal planning can be outsourced to catering companies or family members who are willing to do so. The more you have in the freezer, the less you will worry about when the baby has arrived. You may also not always be there to physically cook for your partner; therefore, she should have the option to defrost whatever is in the freezer and feed herself. People rarely think about meal planning when they're preparing for the baby, but it is very essential as it removes a time-consuming chore from your plate. Time saved on meal planning can be used to bond with your newborn.

What's Happening to Baby

At 32 weeks your baby is now 4 pounds and they are almost ready for life outside of the safety of the uterus. The bones are fully formed, but they have not yet hardened. The baby's lungs are in their final developmental stages and are almost ready to function. The baby may also have hair on their head. Coming in at the size of a pineapple, your baby at 33 weeks is almost 17 inches and weighs around 4.5 pounds. They are continuing to gain weight as they get closer to the 34-week mark. The baby is kicking, and kicking hard. Their senses are able to observe their environment and they continue to sleep. Your baby can see and their pupils are able to dilate and constrict.

At 34 weeks your baby is just over 12 inches long from crown to rump and weighs 5 pounds. The vernix coating has been thickening up until now and it is flaking off into the amniotic fluid. When the baby swallows these pieces of vernix, it helps them develop the use of their stomach and intestines. Now the baby is referred to as "late preterm"; if they are born during this stage, they may have difficulty feeding or breathing, or even be afflicted by jaundice. Fortunately, survival rate is over 99% and the risk of disability is at a low 5%.

When your baby reaches 35 weeks, they will be 5.5 pounds and 12.5 inches long from crown to rump. Although your baby may look fully developed once they reach 35 weeks, there are still some internal developments that need to take place. It is only in the last four to five weeks that the brain goes through a growth spurt. It is estimated that your baby gains half a pound in each week from this point forward, which aids in them growing more fat beneath their skin. The baby's skin is likely to become much less wrinkled at this stage.

What's Happening to Mom

32 weeks may bring more breast leakage, which can be countered by your partner using nursing pads. Braxton Hicks contractions can intensify at this point. You and your partner should know the difference between Braxton Hicks and preterm labor signs. Braxton Hicks contractions have no particular rhythm and disappear as fast as they appear. They do not intensify in pain, or occur closer and closer together. Preterm labor, on the other hand, causes regular contractions that get more intense the longer they occur. If you or your partner are unsure, then the prudent thing to do is to visit your nearest health care facility.

At 33 weeks your partner may be getting tired of being pregnant. She is getting more uncomfortable as the days pass. A change in her body that you may not be able to notice is that her body has produced more blood. Her blood volume may be 40% higher than normal and the heart is pumping much faster in order to accommodate this change. Sometimes her heart may skip a beat, but if it is happening frequently, it is best to inform the doctor. At 34 weeks the symptoms remain relatively the same.

Your partner should consider perineal massage at this point in order to increase the elasticity of the perineum. This is the area between the vagina and the anus that can tear or be cut during delivery if it is not stretching adequately. Your partner may also receive the Tdap vaccine between 27 and 36 weeks. Headaches are common in pregnancy, but they usually bother women in the first and last trimesters, which means your partner may be experiencing them again at 35 weeks. Make sure that she is getting enough sleep while she can. If your baby is measuring big, you and your partner may have to consider giving birth via cesarean section.

What You Should Do

Consider making spreadsheets or having a binder that contains all the plans that you have drawn out for your partner and the baby. Making plans is pointless if you cannot locate those plans at the drop of a hat.

This binder should be located on a coffee table in the home or at a place that is easily accessible for anyone who may need to refer to it. If you want to take a babymoon, this is the time to plan it.

If this is your first child, you may want to spend some time with your partner before things change. If you have other children, this could be the opportunity for you and your partner to be alone and bond over this new baby that is coming. Your partner can barely reach her private parts; therefore, also consider the fact that you are the only one who will be administering perineal massage. Talk to your healthcare provider on how to do this effectively on a daily basis.

What You Should Not Do

Do not assume that you still have time. Your time has run out. The baby could be here at any moment. Wrap up all your preparation plans and memorize them accordingly. Do not leave it to the last day, but rather have one or two run-throughs where you and your partner practice what should happen if she should go into labor. Practice runs are often humorous and enjoyable, because there is no pressure in that situation. Provide constructive criticism to your partner and be receptive to it as well on how you performed or how she performed during the practice run. Take note of what the both of you can do better.

By the end of 35 weeks, you will have just under four weeks to go until your baby's expected due date. Your partner may be reaching her breaking point because her mental health and physical capabilities are stretched to the limit at the moment. If your baby were to be born at this point, then they would have a higher likelihood to survive without any serious complications, as long as they receive the medical interventions that they need. The prognosis would be a positive one.

If you are losing patience with your partner or they are getting snappy with you, then that is also normal, since she is likely frustrated and maybe even a little miserable, depending on her pregnancy symptoms. Try to give her things to do that will cheer her up and put her back into a positive mindset. Sometimes she might want to just complain; let her.

It's not always about finding a solution; sometimes you just need you to listen.

The next chapter will celebrate your partner's pregnant form, as well as outline the frustrations your partner may feel now that her body is in the last weeks of a pregnancy. It'll also discuss what you can do as a partner to make her life easier and more relaxed. She probably looks more beautiful than you've ever seen, but she may not feel that way. Keep reminding her what a goddess she is and how powerful her body is because it can grow a baby inside it. Rub her belly and talk to the baby inside; it's only a matter of time until they make their appearance into the world.

Chapter 9
Third Trimester (36–40 weeks)

Your partner has come a long way. She has been pregnant for around eight months and she feels like she wants to get pregnancy over and done with. Some women take to pregnancy like a fish to water, while others struggle. Because pregnancy is a highly personalized journey for each woman, there's no predicting what your partner will experience or how she will feel at this point. The hormones may also lead to mood changes and make the relationship or communication difficult.

These last few weeks need all the patience that you can muster. If you have been feeling frustrated, trust me, she feels twice the amount of frustration you feel. Your baby could be here at any moment; therefore, you should just try to keep your mind in a positive place so that the birth can be a positive experience for you and your partner. Relish the kicks that you can feel through your partner's belly, and make it a regular habit to speak to your baby so it can recognize your voice. These are the last weeks of pregnancy.

The Limitations of a Pregnant Body

Physical Demands in the Workplace

It is possible that your partner may have a physically demanding job. If a woman is pregnant, physical demands increase the risk of a preterm labor, miscarriage, or an injury while pregnant. Physical demands could be anything that includes lifting heavy objects, constantly bending at the waist, or standing up for extended periods of time. If your partner has a job that includes any of these physical demands, then she is at risk.

The reason why physical demands are a cause for concern is that they increase the risks involved in pregnancy. When we speak of physical demands, we are not referring to physical exercise, which is advised for pregnancy. A pregnant woman's body is constantly evolving, and her hormones can change the state of her joints and ligaments in the spine in order to accommodate the growing uterus. These changes make a pregnant woman highly prone to injuries to her musculoskeletal form, even before she begins to show.

As a pregnant woman's belly expands, this can shift her center of gravity, as discussed in a previous chapter. This change can create an imbalance that can affect her negatively. This increases the chance of her falling and injuring herself. Physical demands at work are linked to menstrual disorders, which are known to reduce the fertility of women.

The typical jobs that can involve physical demands include the following:

- workers in the manufacturing field
- nurses, doctors, and healthcare workers
- flight attendants
- service workers
- workers at a construction site
- firefighters
- law enforcement officers
- farmworkers

- teachers and childcare providers

When your partner finds out that they are pregnant, they should tell their employer immediately so that they can make the necessary accommodations for them. Immediately stop bending, squatting, or stooping; your partner should not lift heavy objects if they are on the floor, or if lifting requires them to bend or reach. Your partner should refrain from reaching or lifting overhead; they should not stand continuously for three hours or more. If the physical demands cannot be avoided, then your partner should sit down regularly and take breaks when she sees fit.

Travel

When your partner is far along in pregnancy, traveling may create some concerns. During the third trimester, your partner may have increased risk of infection, pregnancy complications such as miscarriage and still-birth, and she may have an increased risk of blood clots due to sitting for a long time. The best way to prevent these complications is to avoid long airplane flights and car trips. If the travel is unavoidable, it is suggested that your partner should have enough leg room to stretch, and perhaps walk about every hour or two.

Flying is not recommended at all if your pregnancy is high-risk. Airlines do not allow women after a certain period of gestation because there is a possibility that they give birth unexpectedly on the flight. It is important before you travel to check with the airline if your partner will be allowed on board. She should avoid drinking unpurified water or unpasteurized milk, as well as anything that looks dodgy.

Using a seatbelt is normal if you are in a vehicle. Pregnant women should never forego their seatbelt just because it is uncomfortable. It is not encouraged for a pregnant woman to be an unrestrained passenger, as this is extremely dangerous should an automobile accident occur. To customize the belt to be more comfortable around your partner's belly, position the lap portion of the belt below her belly in order to ensure her safety and that of the baby.

Sleep on Her Back

Sleeping on one's back is not recommended for pregnant women in their third trimester. Lying on your back can cause your uterus, which is very large and heavy, to reduce blood flow to the fetus and the uterus. When your partner is in her last four weeks of pregnancy, lying on her back may not feel comfortable at all. It is recommended for pregnant women to lie on their left side if they are sleeping or at rest.

The uterus naturally rotates to the right when a woman is pregnant; therefore, the left side is considered a favorable choice, because it will lean the uterus more toward the center, and thus improve blood flow. It may be more comfortable for your partner's thighs and hips if you place a pillow between her legs. Body pillows that support her back are also recommended.

Everything Is Difficult

When your partner is in the third trimester, everything will be a challenge to her. She will struggle to get up in the morning and get out of bed. She will struggle to put on her clothes, especially her shoes. Walking may present a challenge. She has aches and pains in her back and legs. When she drives, she has a swollen abdomen she has to accommodate, therefore she moves her seat back but may not be able to reach the pedals. Reaching is not recommended, therefore, she may not be able to get anything for herself. Her body has changed in such a way that it makes simple existence challenging.

What's Happening to Baby

At 36 weeks your baby is nearing 13 inches and weighs around 6 pounds. It is possible that your baby's head is now in a downward position facing the cervix in order to get ready to be born. Your baby has an established sleep cycle that will become more developed in these last weeks. Babies born near term at 36 weeks may require a little assistance to survive. They have a survival rate of over 99%, so if your baby is born now, they have a good chance at making it.

By 37 weeks your baby is a whopping 6.5 pounds; they measure just over 17 inches. The baby is born and immediately can suckle its mother; this is because the baby has been practicing in utero. The baby is now able to coordinate in the sucking and then swallowing motion. If your baby is birthed now, it would mean the said baby is considered early term, as their liver, lungs, and brain are still developing.

Lanugo begins to shed at 38 weeks. These fine hairs typically shed in utero before the baby is born, although the shoulders and arms of the baby may have remnants of lanugo. Your baby is now around 18 inches and anywhere between six and ten pounds. The baby's eye color is a strange, dark blue-gray combination that will change with time. Your baby's eye color is influenced by how much melanin your baby will produce. The final eye color may take up to a year to develop.

At 39 weeks your baby is considered full term and may come during this week. Crown to rump length is at 14 inches and the baby may be around 7.5 pounds in weight. The baby has gained enough fat in order to aid in body temperature regulation. All of their organs are fully formed and the baby is able to exist without medical intervention outside the uterus. In spite of this, the baby's brain and lungs are still developing.

The antibodies that pass to your baby during pregnancy have prepared its immune system for life outside of the womb. These antibodies are needed in order to fight off infections and illnesses. The placenta is responsible for passing antibodies from your partner to the fetus. This is what your baby will use to fight any attacks on its immune system shortly after it is born. If your baby is born via the vagina, the bacteria that enters its nose, mouth, and eyes during birth will also jumpstart its immune response. Colostrum is also filled with antibodies to reinforce your baby's immune system.

40 weeks is the milestone that you have been waiting for for the past nine months. The baby is around 8 pounds in weight and 15 inches from crown to rump. The weight and height that your baby is born at is dependent on various factors, but they are now considered full term and should

be born around this time. By now, the baby looks exactly as a newborn should look. It doesn't matter how their appearance is when they are born, because it is likely that you will not see any imperfection. You will fall in love at first sight with your baby regardless of what they look like.

What's Happening to Mom

At 36 weeks your partner may experience lightening. This happens when the baby changes its position and drops into the mom's pelvis. Don't panic if your partner's belly suddenly looks different than what you're used to. Because the baby has moved lower in her abdomen, this may relieve your partner's shortness of breath. Unfortunately, this lightening will intensify the pressure in the pelvic area.

This drop of the fetus does not mean that your partner is nearing labor or that she is in labor. Lightening can happen anytime from two to four weeks before a woman gives birth. For mothers who have had a child before, this can happen much later, or during labor. To relieve pelvic pain or pressure, the following can alleviate the discomfort your partner feels: a pelvic support belt, elevating your partner's feet when she sits, and taking a warm bath.

By 37 weeks there is an increase in Braxton Hicks contractions and your partner may feel them as often as every 10 to 20 minutes. From this point forward, your partner may lose pieces of their mucus plug in preparation for giving birth. If a considerable chunk of the mucus plug comes out, your partner should let the healthcare provider know at her next appointment. This is not a sign that labor is near, as it may occur days or weeks later.

If your partner is not already waddling, she may begin at 38 weeks when her body has become very large, awkward, and uncomfortable. A myriad of things is happening, such as carrying the extra weight that your partner has gained, accommodating the large uterus in her abdomen, and tolerating increased pressure in her pelvic area. The graceful beauty that you impregnated may not be as graceful as clumsiness takes the lead. Her center of gravity is off and her joints and ligaments have loosened up in preparation for childbirth; therefore, she is a little unstable and prone to falling.

Your partner's body is preparing itself for the miracle of birth. The pressure of the baby's head descending lower and lower into the pelvis prepares her cervix to soften and shorten. This is called effacement, or ripening of the cervix. At some point, the cervix has to begin to dilate for the baby to come out. Dilation can happen gradually over a few weeks, or quickly during labor. The hormonal prostaglandins can help the cervix get ready for the birth of your baby, but they can also cause loose stools. Diarrhea is expected during this time.

It is normal that, even after the 40 weeks milestone has elapsed, a woman still does not go into labor. If this is her first child, she may go into labor anytime after 41 weeks. The due date is estimated because pregnancy is unpredictable. Babies come on their own schedule. Be prepared for the labor signs to begin at any moment. There is no way to predict what kind of labor your partner will have, but you should be prepared for anything. Some women have quick and easy labor, and others have a slow, painful experience. You'll know where she falls when it begins.

What You Should Do

If the baby stops moving at any point or it is moving less frequently, keep track of those movements. Give your partner something to eat and allow her to lay down on her left side. Keep track of your baby's movements for an hour and you should reach around 10 movements. If these movements are significantly less, then your partner should consult her doctor on what she is observing.

Learn how to count contractions or download an app that can help you keep track when everything begins. A lot of parents will take time off after the baby is born, but it may be beneficial if you take a little time off before the baby is born as well in order to put the final touches on your preparation. There are some activities that you can partake in that may encourage your partner's body to begin laboring. These tips may become helpful if your partner becomes overdue.

Walking is an upright motion that encourages the baby to descend further into the pelvis. You could try stimulating your partner's nipples, as nipple play encourages the release of oxytocin, which will stimulate contractions. It is also believed that having sex will encourage labor, as there are prostaglandins in semen. Oxytocin is released during an orgasm, which is also helpful to stimulate labor.

What You Should Not Do

Internal exams, where the healthcare provider monitors cervix for dilation, may begin during this phase. You may have to get used to your partner being checked internally numerous times. When she goes into labor, she will be checked on how far her cervix has effaced almost on an hourly basis. Depending on your level of maturity, they might make you feel uncomfortable. It may be a little awkward watching a healthcare provider poking around your partner's genitals. Don't get too uncomfortable about it, because it's going to happen a lot. They're trying to help your partner and that's the only way that they can.

When you notice that your partner has begun nesting, do not let her do everything on her own. Nesting can include activities like cooking, cleaning, shopping, getting supplies, and preparing the nursery. The baby requires very little when it is brought home from the hospital, but is it necessary for you to join in the nesting activities. This is also a good time to seek advice from other parents if you are experiencing insecurity about getting in the way during labor, or how you may feel when your partner is in pain. Do not bottle up these concerns, but rather seek advice from other parents and medical health professionals.

The following chapters will be about the birth of your baby and how to prepare for that. The way they depict a woman's labor in the movies is very erroneous, therefore, do not expect anything like that. Giving birth is miraculous and spectacular. The human body knows how to cope and compensate when it is in pain. You don't have to worry, because your partner's body was designed to give birth. It may be unpleasant feeling helpless and not being able to directly help, but with every contraction, know that your baby is closer to being in your arms.

Chapter 10
Birth

The momentous day has arrived when you will meet your baby. This is the moment that you and your partner have been daydreaming about for the past 40+ weeks or less. It can happen in so many different ways. My job is to sensitize you to all the different ways that your partner can give birth. You may be feeling anxious, afraid, and unsure; your partner is feeling the same way. If this is her first time giving birth, she is protected by the naïveté of being a new mom. My wife was much more anxious the second time around.

There is no guarantee that everything will work out fine. Although the possibility is low, it is possible that you may lose the baby during birth or that it may be a stillbirth. There is also a risk of maternal death, although that is not a common occurrence. A majority of the time, things will go well, but it is important to take it one step at a time. Whatever coping methods that you have you should lean on at this time. If you are a spiritual or religious person, now is the time to pray.

All the Different Ways a Woman Can Give Birth

Until 75 years ago, women labored and gave birth at home. Women labored in the old time without any interference or invasive monitoring methods. This changed the more medicine evolved. Interventions to reduce maternal deaths inevitably led to more invasive monitoring during birth. Some people still prefer to labor and birth their babies at home without too much interference from medical professionals. Giving birth is a special time and your partner should be as comfortable as possible.

Your partner's birth story is influenced by various things, such as the delivery options and location. Before you decide on which method to use, all the risks and benefits of each should be weighed by you and your partner in order to determine what is right for her. Medical advancements have made it so that annually less than 600 women die in the US from complications during birth.

Although the level of pain varies from woman to woman, it can be agreed that childbirth is painful. In spite of this pain, most women recover quickly and the pain is short-lived. Being pregnant doesn't mean she will have to suffer through the pain of childbirth if she feels that she is not able to do so. There are always ways women can reduce the amount of pain they feel during childbirth, naturally or not.

Unassisted Childbirth

A woman who desires to birth her child unassisted is often taught how to handle that situation by attending classes and learning how she needs to be prepared. She will also be guided on what she should expect. It is in these classes that she will learn about the stages of labor and how to use breathing techniques to relax and reduce the intensity of the pain. What is discussed during these classes is what will happen to the vagina during birth and afterward. The classes also cover how to care for a newborn in the initial days.

Home Birth

Some women choose a home birth because of the safe and relaxing environment that their home provides them. This kind of birthing method is only available for those women who fall into the low-risk pregnancy category. Home births are vaginal deliveries that do not involve the administration of medication to reduce the pain of childbirth. Instead, they utilize some techniques that are said to promote easier labor and reduce childbirth pain.

Home births are attended to by a midwife or a doula; both are certified professionals that usually work in birthing centers and are equipped and able to assist a laboring woman. The advantages of home births include not needing a transport to and from the hospital after giving birth; anyone can be invited to attend the birth of the baby; the comfort of home means that they have snacks and other comforts available; and they can recover quite easily while transitioning from birth to nursing. Being in their home environment makes women more comfortable to grunt or yell or make any other noise that they want to during labor.

There are some disadvantages that come with having a home birth. If there is any special equipment desired during labor, it has to be set up in advance. If the home is located in a remote area or the midwife has to travel in bad weather, it may be difficult for them to have access to the home. If complications arise at home, they will need to transport the laboring woman to the hospital. Some women are not comfortable with birthing at home, as medical care is not very close should things go wrong.

Vaginal Delivery (With or Without Medication)

Vaginal delivery is a way a mother labors and gives birth to a baby via the vagina. The benefits of this kind of delivery are that there is a lower rate of infection in women who deliver in this way, and their hospital stays are usually much shorter. Mothers who give birth vaginally, with or without medication, recover much more quickly compared to those who give birth via C-section. Infants that are born vaginally will have less respiratory problems than their counterparts who are born via surgery.

This is one of the most celebrated ways to birth a child, but it doesn't come without disadvantages. A vaginal birth may cause a woman's perineum to tear during the delivery; the degree of the tear, or how severe it is, is unpredictable in every scenario. That is why doctors often perform an episiotomy if they can see that the perineum is not stretching adequately. An episiotomy is controlled, and therefore, there is less risk of the cut reaching the anus. Unfortunately, not everybody has the luxury of giving birth vaginally, and some women are prohibited from doing so due to medical reasons.

Water Birth

When a woman chooses to have a water birth, she can go through all the stages of labor and birth in a birthing tub. She may also choose to carry out a majority of her labor in the tub and then move to a different position outside of the tub in order to deliver the baby. It is possible for the baby to be delivered underwater. This kind of birth is said to be more relaxing, as the water alleviates some of the pain of childbirth. Birthing tubs may be found in birthing centers and certain hospitals. Portable tubs may be brought into the home for a homebirth.

The benefits of a water birth are that being in the water provides a more relaxed and less painful environment to labor in, and the woman is free to change her positions as she wishes in order to be more comfortable. With a water birth, a woman has the freedom to move into a variety of positions that may feel more natural to her. A woman's partner can provide her more comfort and support during a water birth by getting into the tub with her.

The disadvantage of a water birth is, as its critics state, that there is an increased risk of infection; the tub and water itself need to be clean and fresh to minimize these risks. If the water birth is not taking place in a birthing center or hospital where the tubs are already set up, then there needs to be some logistical planning involved with setting up the tub at the birthing location, as well as warming the water that will fill the tub. If complications arise, the woman will have to be transported to a hospital timeously.

Hospital Delivery

Giving birth in a hospital allows a woman almost the same courtesies as a home birth except that at the hospital, if something goes wrong, then there are doctors on the court to intervene surgically if need be. A woman can choose to give birth with or without medication. Nowadays, a woman can also opt to go straight for a C-section if she sees fit instead of it being an emergency intervention. Hospital births have become the norm as compared to birthing at home.

The benefits of a hospital delivery include having access to specialized medical interventions in cases of emergency. A woman's life, and that of the baby, can be saved much more easily when they have quicker access to specialized care. High-risk pregnancies or births can be monitored much more closely with a variety of special devices and machines. A woman who gives birth in a hospital has an array of options when it comes to pain management, including gas and epidural or pethidine.

The negative risks of birthing in a hospital include that the medical caregivers can intervene, even if the woman doesn't want said interventions. A woman can be rushed through the various stages of labor, which could increase the likelihood of her receiving an episiotomy or a cesarean. There is a risk of infection when one is admitted in a hospital, and this also applies when a woman is giving birth.

Forceps Delivery

In order to facilitate a forceps-assisted delivery, curved instruments are inserted into the birth canal to grip onto the infant and pull them out. If the baby is in a breech position, this kind of delivery cannot be put to use. Forceps delivery is advantageous when a woman has become too exhausted to push the baby out, or if they need to be delivered faster than what is naturally possible.

Vacuum Extraction

Sometimes a woman is not able to complete her natural birth and may need to receive medical assistance. A vacuum-assisted delivery occurs when the baby is in the birth canal and a soft cup is attached to the head of the baby, while the person delivering the baby is holding a pump that will suction the baby out of the canal. An advantage of a vacuum extraction is that the baby is in distress for a shorter amount of time than during a C-section delivery. Because the suction cup is attached to the head of the baby, there is a risk that they will experience some kind of scalp trauma, or even bleeding on or in the head.

C-Section

When a woman is unable to give birth naturally, she will be assisted to birth her baby. Pregnancy can come with all kinds of complications. Sometimes the intervention of the doctors is necessary to save the life of both the mom and the baby. In the United States, a third of all births are delivered via C-section. The World Health Organization states that the C-section rate should be at 10–15% in the United States, but that the rate is much higher because of overuse and the high occurrence of elective C-sections.

A C-section is a surgery where a small horizontal incision is made in the lower abdomen; the baby is then delivered through this incision. A mom who delivers her baby by C-section, and experiences no complications, is expected to stay three days in the hospital. Recovery takes eight weeks. An advantage of a C-section is that it can be planned ahead of time and scheduled months in advance. C-sections carry a risk of infection, because it is surgery. Your stitches can rupture or get infected.

What's Happening to Mom

There are three stages of labor that your partner will experience. Early labor, active labor, and transition constitutes the first stage; the second stage is when your partner is pushing and the baby is birthed; the third stage includes the delivery of the placenta.

Early Labor

Uterine contractions kickstart early labor. Depending on the woman, they can either be irregular and not very painful, usually lasting only up to 45 seconds at a time, or they can be quite painful from the beginning. You know your partner is in early labor when she has a bloody show or her water breaks. With every contraction, your partner's cervix is effacing and dilating. Braxton Hicks will usually let up if you change positions, but contractions do not stop; this stage can last up to two days, but it is important to let your healthcare provider know what is happening to your partner. A lot of women prefer to get through early labor at home.

Active Labor

When your partner's cervix has dilated three or more centimeters, she is said to be in active labor. The cervix may dilate 1 cm per hour. During this stage, the contractions occur regularly and more often; they also become stronger and more painful. As the labor progresses, they will happen closer together and become much more painful. The baby is steadily moving toward the birth canal. It is at this point that your partner should be in the place that she wishes to give birth. "You aren't in established labor until your contractions arrive at a steady rate and consistently increase in both intensity and duration" (Weiss, 2022).

In order to keep track of your partner's contractions, you should mark the time when the contraction is beginning, then mark when it ends. Note how long the contraction lasted and then also note when the next one begins. You will know it's time to get to the hospital or birthing center when your partner's contractions are 45 seconds or longer and occur every three to five minutes. Technology is there to help you; there are apps you can use to time your partner's contractions so that you have them recorded if you need to let their healthcare provider know what is going on.

Transition

Transition constitutes the conclusion of the first stage of labor. It is the shortest part, but also the most difficult. The contractions are often very intense and can last up to two minutes. The time between contractions is short, so women do not have time to recover from the last contraction. The cervix is open to its widest point, and it is at this time that the woman may vomit or feel nauseous, because she is at the peak of the pain. Shivering and dizziness are not uncommon. When your partner has reached 10 cm the second stage of labor can begin. She will feel immense pressure and an urge to push; if she has had an epidural, then these sensations will be dulled.

Delivery

When a woman has reached the point of pushing, she will feel an urge that is similar to when she has to move her bowels. Each push will slowly move the baby down the birth canal toward the entrance of the vagina. When the baby's head has emerged from your partner's vagina and remains visible, this is when the baby is said to be crowning; if at this stage the baby's head is still slipping back inside, then they are not yet crowning. The head is the hardest part to deliver and the healthcare provider will guide the baby out while also checking that the cord has not slipped around the baby's neck. This stage will come to an end with the birth of your long-awaited baby.

Placenta

The final stage of labor constitutes delivering the placenta. This usually happens within 30 minutes of labor. Your partner may feel some contractions and the urge to push again. Once the placenta is delivered, then your partner's labor is complete.

What's Happening to Baby

When a baby is born at full term, they could measure anywhere from 17 to 22 inches. Moreover, their weight could be between 5.5–10 pounds. Their appearance may be somewhat shocking to you. Birth can be somewhat traumatic for a baby and there may be some signs of that experience showing on the baby. Being born vaginally and having a soft skull may mean the baby's head comes out cone-shaped. This will resolve itself after a few days.

Lanugo and vernix may still cover the baby's skin and their eyes could be swollen. Their hands and feet may have a blue tone to them while baby's genitals may appear swollen. Your baby may have white spots or a rash, or some kind of acne. Give the baby time and they'll settle in and begin to look more and more like those babies in the magazines.

Tests/Procedures

After the baby is born, there will be a few tests that will either be done on the baby right away or that will be done in the coming days. Your baby's APGAR score will be measured within five minutes of your baby being born and can be performed while your baby is on your partner's chest. The birthing staff will assess the baby's heart rate, muscle tone, reflexes, respiratory effort, and their skin color. The reason why this test may happen on your partner's chest is because, right after the baby is born, the doctor will suction amniotic fluid and mucus out of your baby's nose and mouth, dry the baby, and place them on your partner's stomach or chest so that they can have skin-to-skin contact. If the baby is showing signs of distress, then they will likely assess the baby before bringing it to you.

The umbilical cord will be cut either by you or the healthcare provider, and this will separate the baby from the placenta, which has provided nourishment from around 13 weeks' gestation. If you are present in the room when your partner gives birth, this is an honor that is often given to fathers. The baby's weight will be taken, as well as their length; these measurements will be taken again at each medical appointment as the baby is growing. There will be an ointment or eye drops called erythromycin antibiotic applied to the baby's eyes to prevent infection from the germs that they may have contracted during birth. If your baby is a boy and you decide this is the best course of action, they may be circumcised at birth. Circumcision may be delayed for religious reasons, such as in the Jewish faith where circumcision is delayed for eight days and is done at a special ceremony.

Vitamin K is administered to the baby within six hours so that the baby's risk of brain and other bleeding is reduced, as this injection promotes proper blood clotting. It is recommended that the first dose of the hepatitis B vaccine is given to a newborn within 24 hours of birth.

The baby may also receive a hearing test. A screening test called a PKU test may be administered within two days, where the baby's heel is pricked to collect drops of blood so that the healthcare provider may test for 50 different illnesses that include congenital hypothyroidism, galactosemia, and phenylketonuria.

What You Should Do

If your partner is with you, you can help her to encourage labor by going for walks with her, stimulating her nipples, and engaging in sexual intercourse that allows your semen to reach her cervix. Try to enjoy the last few moments that you have with your partner and your family before everything changes. Go over all the preparation and make sure that everything is ready to go. Have a poker face so that when your partner is feeling anxious or scared, you are there to reassure her, even if you are also scared. Make sure your support system or the people you lean on for support are on standby. Your partner will lean on you and you will lean on them.

What You Should Not Do

Do not freak out. There is a lot of comedy surrounding fathers who faint in the delivery room; this is because they have no idea what is in store for them when they are present during their child's birth. Watch as many birthing videos as you can so that you are somewhat prepared for what you will witness. It is a little gruesome because there can be a lot of blood. Keep calm and relax.

With the birth of your baby, you will have successfully completed the pregnancy process and will be moving toward your journey as a father. Whether or not this is your first baby, there is something special about having a new human in your home. That precious baby smell and the little cooing sounds they make makes it all worthwhile. Your partner may have gained a new respect from you as you recall what she has gone through. Well done to you both!

Conclusion

Being a father is one of the most rewarding things in my life; you will soon understand why. The first few days after the baby is born are the most serene. Your partner is likely tired from giving birth and is trying to rest as much as possible, while your baby is settling into the new environment outside the womb. You and your partner are getting to know your baby, and they are getting to know you, too. After your partner and your baby are discharged and you are home, it may feel awkward trying to figure out what your role is, especially if your partner is able to breastfeed.

Although your partner may seem like she has recovered, she has to go through postpartum care and likely nurse her perineum or C-section scar. When you can take the baby and give your partner a rest, please do so; try to help with all household chores, such as your partner's and the baby's laundry, as well as cleaning out their room regularly. Prepare all your partner's meals and bring them to her room so that she doesn't need to get out of bed.

Your baby will likely have the same schedule they had in utero, sleeping and waking at a similar time as they did when your partner was still pregnant. You and your partner will have to give the baby care and adapt your own schedules around theirs. The newborn phase is like the honeymoon phase; your baby is likely to sleep most of the time and feed every two hours or so. This is a whole new adventure for you and them; enjoy every moment that you can, because the time flies quite quickly.

Postpartum Depression

Due to the fluctuating hormones that your partner may experience after giving birth, she may experience "baby blues." This is characterized by crying spells, mood swings, anxiety, and mild insomnia. A lot of women go through this, and it may affect your partner, too. The baby blues may begin from two days postpartum and last for up to two weeks. Postpartum depression can affect new moms; postpartum psychosis is rare, but it is a mood disorder that can develop after birth. If any of these affect your partner, she should not be ashamed, as there is nothing that she has done wrong.

Symptoms of postpartum depression include crying, severe mood swings, inability to bond with the baby, excessive eating or loss of appetite, insomnia, and withdrawing from loved ones, to name a few. Your partner may have to seek help if her symptoms are getting worse, they are not fading after a couple of weeks, she is unable to care for herself or the baby, and is having suicidal thoughts or thoughts of harming the baby.

You Have a Bond

Look back at the journey you have been on with your partner and the baby, even before it got here. You were there through the initial intense pregnancy symptoms of the first trimester. You held your partner's hair as she retched into the bowl of the toilet. You were there when the ultrasound revealed the sex of the baby. When your partner felt the first kicks, you were just as excited as she was to feel them. When her labor began, you were both riddled with anxiety. There are things you know that no one else does; you feel that thing that ties you all together.

Take over with the baby, not only to give your partner a rest, but also to establish your bond. You spent countless hours conversing with the baby when it was still in the womb. Continue to speak to your baby and reassure it that you are there to offer protection, love, and guidance. Take off your shirt and have some skin-to-skin bonding time with your baby so that you can reinforce your bond. When the baby can recognize your voice and how you smell, they will 'know' who you are.

All the things you did for your partner when she was pregnant, and what you continue to do for her now that she has given birth, is a testament to the love you have for her and your baby. As the primary caregiver for the baby, you should recognize that her well-being is vital for the well-being of your baby. She cannot be a good mother if she does not feel okay. The same is true for you. You are unable to care for your family if you are also not feeling fine.

Find some alone time with your partner, so that you can let her know how proud of her you are that she managed to give birth to a whole baby. She might be feeling quite exhausted and emotionally drained, but it is important to let her know that she has done an amazing job. Find time alone with your baby and feed or change it; read your baby bedtime stories or sing while rocking on a rocking chair. You may not be able to toss a pig skin yet, but you can do little things to show your love for the baby.

Treat Yourself

You have been the backbone of support for your entire family. Now that the baby is here, you can take some time to treat yourself for the job you continue to do. Whether it's a new haircut or a half-body deep stone massage, find time to replenish yourself. Your mental well-being is crucial to the success of the family; if you need to step away to rejuvenate yourself, then do so. If you need help, seek it from your family or from health care providers. Fathers can be affected by postpartum depression, too. Your role is as important as your partner's role as the mother of the baby. The baby will forever be grateful to you for all the effort you have put into their well-being. Congratulations! You are now a dad!

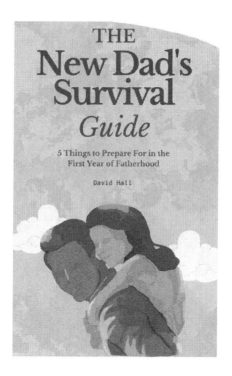

Dear reader,

Thank you for choosing to read my book. I hope you found it informative and thought-provoking. If you enjoyed the book and found it helpful, I would be grateful if you could take a few moments to leave a review on Amazon.

Your feedback and thoughts are important to me as an author and can help others decide if this book is right for them. It would be wonderful to hear your opinion, whether positive or negative, and any suggestions you may have for future editions.

Thank you for your time and consideration. Happy reading!

Bibliography

American Pregnancy Association. (2021, April 27). *Miscarriage: Signs, symptoms, treatment and prevention.* American Pregnancy Association. https://americanpregnancy.org/getting-pregnant/pregnancy-loss/signs-of-miscarriage/

Babylist. (2022, May 9). *Everything you need to pack in your hospital bag.* Babylist. https://www.babylist.com/hello-baby/what-to-pack-in-your-hospital-bag

Bjarnadottir, A. (2018, July 18). *11 foods and beverages to avoid during pregnancy.* Healthline. https://www.healthline.com/nutrition/11-foods-to-avoid-during-pregnancy

Brazier, Y. (2020, October 25). *Puberty in boys and girls: What is it all about?* Medical News Today. https://www.medicalnewstoday.com/articles/156451

Cadman, B. (2019, February 22). *What to know about sex during pregnancy.* Medical News Today. https://www.medicalnewstoday.com/articles/321648#benefits

Centers For Disease Control And Prevention. (2020, July 9). *Physical demands.* Centers for Disease Control and Prevention. https://www.cdc.gov/niosh/topics/repro/physicaldemands.html

Daley, K. (2018, December 19). *How pregnancy hormones affect your body in each trimester.* Today's Parent. https://www.todaysparent.com/pregnancy/pregnancy-health/how-pregnancy-hormones-affect-your-body-in-each-trimester/

Danielsson, K. (2008, August 13). *What is fetal viability?* Verywell Family. https://www.verywellfamily.com/premature-birth-and-viability-2371529

Dugas, C., & Slane, V. H. (2019, May 11). *Miscarriage.* National Center for Biotechnology Information. https://www.ncbi.nlm.nih.gov/books/NBK532992/

Gurevich, R. (2021, June 17). *Facts about predicting the sex of your baby.* Verywell Family. https://www.verywellfamily.com/predicting-the-sex-of-your-baby-4580299

Holland, K. (2020, October 13). *28 weeks pregnant: What you need to know.* Healthline. https://www.healthline.com/health/pregnancy/28-weeks-pregnant?utm_source=ReadNext#your-baby

Knapp, J. (2022, April 22). *Your pregnancy to-do list.* Parents. https://www.parents.com/pregnancy/week-by-week/your-pregnancy-to-do-list/

Marcin, A., & Crider, C. (2022, March 29). *20 weeks pregnant: Baby size, symptoms, checklist & tips.* Healthline. https://www.healthline.com/health/pregnancy/20-weeks-pregnant?utm_source=ReadNext#20-week-scan

Mayo Clinic. (2018, September 1). *Postpartum depression - symptoms and causes.* Mayo Clinic. https://www.mayoclinic.org/diseases-conditions/postpartum-depression/symptoms-causes/syc-20376617

McDermott, A. (2017a, October 23). *18 weeks pregnant: Symptoms, tips, and more.* Healthline. https://www.healthline.com/health/pregnancy/18-weeks-pregnant

McDermott, A. (2017b, October 23). *21 weeks pregnant: Symptoms, tips, and more.* Healthline. https://www.healthline.com/health/pregnancy/21-weeks-pregnant?utm_source=ReadNext#symptoms

Bibliography

NHS. (2020, December 1). *How to make a birth plan*. NHS. https://www.nhs.uk/pregnancy/labour-and-birth/preparing-for-the-birth/how-to-make-a-birth-plan/

Oberg, E. (2018). *Childbirth types: Natural childbirth, water birth, home birth*. Medicine-Net. https://www.medicinenet.com/7_childbirth_and_delivery_methods/article.htm

Pevzner, H. (2019). *Week 34 of your pregnancy*. Verywell Family. https://www.verywellfamily.com/34-weeks-pregnant-4159227

Pevzner, H. (2021a, June 14). *Week 3 of your pregnancy*. Verywell Family. https://www.verywellfamily.com/3-weeks-pregnant-4158839

Pevzner, H. (2021b, June 14). *Week 4 of your pregnancy*. Verywell Family. https://www.verywellfamily.com/4-weeks-pregnant-4158847

Pevzner, H. (2021c, June 14). Week 7 of your pregnancy. Verywell Family. https://www.verywellfamily.com/7-weeks-pregnant-4158916

Pevzner, H. (2021d, June 14). *Week 10 of your pregnancy*. Verywell Family. https://www.verywellfamily.com/10-weeks-pregnant-4158926

Pevzner, H. (2021e, June 14). *Week 11 of your pregnancy*. Verywell Family. https://www.verywellfamily.com/11-weeks-pregnant-4158930

Pevzner, H. (2021f, June 14). *Week 12 of your pregnancy*. Verywell Family. https://www.verywellfamily.com/12-weeks-pregnant-4158934

Pevzner, H. (2021g, June 14). *Week 13 of your pregnancy*. Verywell Family. https://www.verywellfamily.com/13-weeks-pregnant-4158941

Pevzner, H. (2021h, June 14). *Week 17 of your pregnancy*. Verywell Family. https://www.verywellfamily.com/17-weeks-pregnant-4159005

Pevzner, H. (2021i, June 14). *Week 35 of your pregnancy*. Verywell Family. https://www.verywellfamily.com/35-weeks-pregnant-4159237

Pevzner, H. (2021j, June 14). *Week 36 of your pregnancy*. Verywell Family. https://www.verywellfamily.com/36-weeks-pregnant-4159243

Pevzner, H. (2021k, June 14). *Week 37 of your pregnancy*. Verywell Family. https://www.verywellfamily.com/37-weeks-pregnant-4159250

Pevzner, H. (2021l, June 14). *Week 38 of your pregnancy*. Verywell Family. https://www.verywellfamily.com/38-weeks-pregnant-4159251

Pevzner, H. (2021m, June 14). *Week 39 of your pregnancy*. Verywell Family. https://www.verywellfamily.com/39-weeks-pregnant-4159263

Pevzner, H. (2021n, June 14). *Week 40 of your pregnancy*. Verywell Family. https://www.verywellfamily.com/40-weeks-pregnant-4159264

Pevzner, H. (2021o, July 19). *Week 5 of your pregnancy*. Verywell Family. https://www.verywellfamily.com/5-weeks-pregnant-4158868#toc-at-your-doctors-office

Pevzner, H. (2021p, July 19). *Week 6 of your pregnancy*. Verywell Family. https://www.verywellfamily.com/6-weeks-pregnant-4158911

Pevzner, H. (2021q, July 19). *Week 8 of your pregnancy*. Verywell Family. https://www.verywellfamily.com/8-weeks-pregnant-4158920

Pevzner, H. (2021r, July 19). *Week 9 of your pregnancy*. Verywell Family. https://www.verywellfamily.com/9-weeks-pregnant-4158922

Roland, J. (2017a, October 18). *29 weeks pregnant: Symptoms, tips, and more*. Healthline. https://www.healthline.com/health/pregnancy/29-weeks-pregnant?utm_source=ReadNext#your-body

Roland, J. (2017b, October 19). *24 weeks pregnant: Symptoms, tips, and more*. Healthline.

Bibliography

https://www.healthline.com/health/pregnancy/24-weeks-pregnant?utm_source=Read-Next#things-to-do

Roland, J. (2017c, October 23). *16 weeks pregnant: Symptoms, tips, and more.* Healthline. https://www.healthline.com/health/pregnancy/16-weeks-pregnant?utm_source=ReadNext

Roland, J. (2017d, October 23). *19 weeks pregnant: Symptoms, tips, and more.* Healthline. https://www.healthline.com/health/pregnancy/19-weeks-pregnant?utm_source=ReadNext

Roland, J. (2021, August 5). *23 weeks pregnant: Symptoms, tips, and more.* Healthline. https://www.healthline.com/health/pregnancy/23-weeks-pregnant?utm_source=Read-Next#symptoms

Schaeffar, J. (2017, October 18). *30 weeks pregnant: Symptoms, tips, and more.* Healthline. https://www.healthline.com/health/pregnancy/30-weeks-pregnant?utm_source=Read-Next#call-the-doctor

Schaeffer, J. (2017a, October 18). *26 weeks pregnant: Symptoms, tips, and more.* Healthline. https://www.healthline.com/health/pregnancy/26-weeks-pregnant

Schaeffer, J. (2017b, October 23). *14 weeks pregnant: Symptoms, tips, and more.* Healthline. https://www.healthline.com/health/pregnancy/14-weeks-pregnant

Schaeffer, J. (2017c, October 23). *17 weeks pregnant: Symptoms, tips, and more.* Healthline. https://www.healthline.com/health/pregnancy/17-weeks-pregnant?utm_source=ReadNext

Schaeffer, J. (2020, October 6). *22 weeks pregnant: Symptoms, tips, and more.* Healthline. https://www.healthline.com/health/pregnancy/22-weeks-pregnant?utm_source=Read-Next#symptoms

Silver, N. (2017a, October 18). *33 weeks pregnant: Symptoms, tips, and more.* Healthline. https://www.healthline.com/health/pregnancy/33-weeks-pregnant?utm_source=Read-Next#twins

Silver, N. (2017b, October 19). *25 weeks pregnant: Symptoms, tips, and more.* Healthline. https://www.healthline.com/health/pregnancy/25-weeks-pregnant?utm_source=Read-Next#your-body

Silver, N. (2017c, October 23). *15 weeks pregnant: Symptoms, tips, and more.* Healthline. https://www.healthline.com/health/pregnancy/15-weeks-pregnant?utm_source=ReadNext

The Healthline Editorial Team. (2018, December 5). *Third trimester pregnancy: Concerns and tips.* Healthline. https://www.healthline.com/health/pregnancy/third-trimester-concerns-tips#hospital-stay

UCSF Health. (n.d.). *Conception: How It Works.* UCSF Health. https://www.ucsfhealth.org/education/conception-how-it-works

Viarenich, N. (2021, March 11). *Belly expansion during pregnancy: What to expect.* Flo Health. https://flo.health/pregnancy/pregnancy-health/staying-healthy/belly-expansion#:~:text=First%2Dtime%20mothers%20can%20expect

Weiss, R. E. (2020, December 1). *What Is Implantation Bleeding?* Verywell Family. https://www.verywellfamily.com/am-i-having-implantation-bleeding-in-pregnancy-2759953

Weiss, R. E. (2022, January 26). *How do you time contractions during labor?* Verywell Family. https://www.verywellfamily.com/how-to-time-contractions-2752965

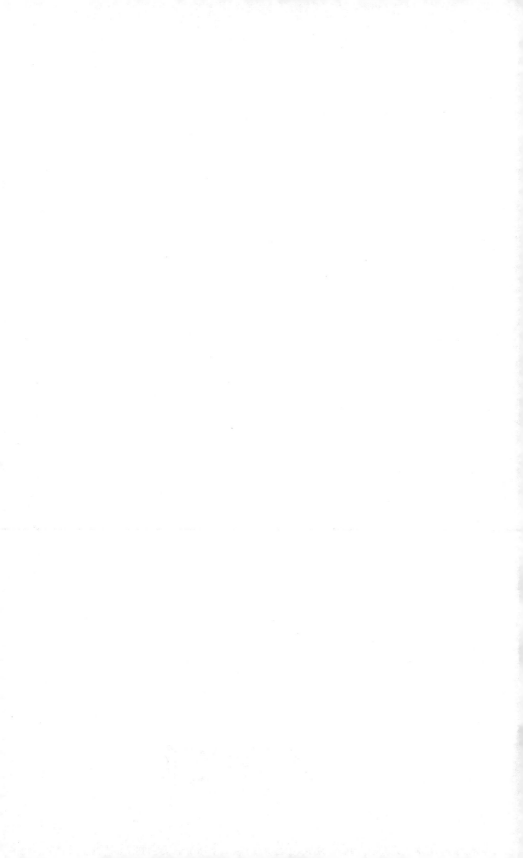

Printed in Great Britain
by Amazon

35875807R00059